Epidermal Ce

MW01106601

Epidermal Cell Tumors: The Basics

Bruce R. Smoller

Department of Pathology
University of Arkansas for Medical Sciences
Little Rock, AR, USA

and

Kim M. Hiatt

Department of Pathology
University of Arkansas for Medical Sciences
Little Rock, AR, USA

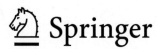 Springer

Bruce R. Smoller
Department of Pathology
University of Arkansas for
  Medical Sciences
Little Rock, AR 72205, USA

Kim M. Hiatt
Department of Pathology
University of Arkansas for
  Medical Sciences
Little Rock, AR 72205, USA

ISBN 978-1-4419-7703-8   e-ISBN 978-1-4419-7704-5
DOI 10.1007/978-1-4419-7704-5
Springer New York Dordrecht Heidelberg London

Springer is part of Springer Science+Business Media (www.springer.com)

Preface

This book represents the third volume in our series on basic dermatopathology. Like the others, this hopes to provide a framework for the conceptualization of epithelial-based tumors. The small size is intentional in attempting to provide an easy-to-use reference atlas to keep within reach of the daily sign-out. This volume of the series is devoted to epidermal- and dermal-based tumors of epithelial origin. We aim to reach medical students, pathology residents, dermatology residents, and surgical pathologists. Accordingly, the content is thorough, but not meant to be comprehensive. Each entity is accompanied by brief clinical notes, a description of the most common histologic findings, and an atlas of photographs.

Little Rock, Arkansas

Bruce R. Smoller
Kim M. Hiatt

Acknowledgement

As always, Bruce Smoller wishes to acknowledge his wife, Laura, and two children, Jason and Gabriel, for their constant enthusiastic support and love. And, Dr. Hiatt would like to thank her husband, Jim, for his support and for the enjoyment that her children Stephanie, Nicholas, Kaitlyn, and Natalie continue to bring to each day.

Contents

Chapter 1
Benign Melanocytic Proliferations

- Benign melanocytic proliferations
  - Also known as melanocytic nevi, "moles"
    - "Nevus" means hamartoma and is likely a misnomer and nevi have been shown to be true clonal proliferations
  - Present at birth, but most arise during adolescence or early adulthood
  - Only rarely arise later in life (after age 40)
  - Present in vast majority of Caucasians, also present in other racial groups
  - Potential for malignant transformation is less than 1/100,000 in acquired melanocytic nevi
- Benign melanocytic proliferations (see Table 1.1)
- Common melanocytic nevus
- Proposed life cycle for melanocytic proliferations (including common acquired, congenital, dysplastic or atypical, Spitz, acral)
  - Clinical
    - *Junctional nevus* – flat, deeply pigmented lesions with sharp edges, usually oval or circular
    - *Compound nevus* – raised above surface of skin, retain pigmentation

B.R. Smoller, K.M. Hiatt, *Epidermal Cell Tumors: The Basics*,
DOI 10.1007/978-1-4419-7704-5_1,

Table 1.1 Benign melanocytic proliferations

Common acquired melanocytic nevus	
Congenital melanocytic nevus	
Halo nevus	
Nevus of special sites (acral, genital)	
Combined nevus	
Balloon cell nevus	Volume III, Chapter 3
Spindle and epithelioid cell (Spitz) nevus	Volume III, Chapter 3
Blue nevus	Volume II, Chapter 12

- o *Intradermal nevus* – nodular to polypoid, lose pigment (skin-colored)

– Histologic

- o *Junctional nevus* – proliferation of melanocytes confined to the epidermis, largely nested along basement membrane (Figs. 1.1 and 1.2)
- o *Compound nevus* – some melanocytes drop into dermis and some remain in the epidermis (Fig. 1.3)
- o *Intradermal nevus* – intraepidermal component of melanocytic proliferation is absent; all residual melanocytes are within dermis (Fig. 1.4)

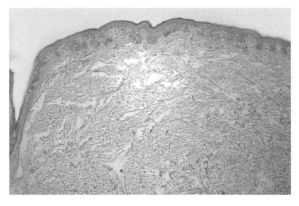

Fig. 1.1 Junctional melanocytic nevus with nests of melanocytes confined to the base of rete ridges. Original magnification ×40

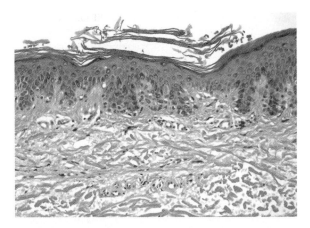

Fig. 1.2 Junctional melanocytic nevus demonstrates small nests of melanocytes that can be differentiated from keratinocytes based upon morphologic features. Original magnification ×200

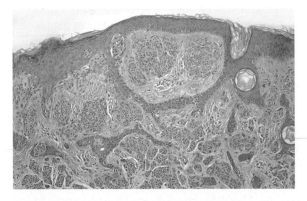

Fig. 1.3 Compound melanocytic nevus has nests of nevus cells within the epidermis as well as within the dermis. Original magnification ×100

- Acquired melanocytic nevus

  - Histologic

    - Junctional component should be almost entirely nested and sharply circumscribed

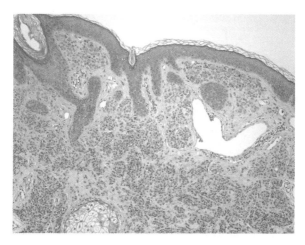

Fig. 1.4 Intradermal nevus demonstrates nests of melanocytes restricted to the dermis with no epidermal involvement. Original magnification ×100

o Proliferation of single melanocytes is uncommon

o "Pagetoid" cells may occur secondary to trauma, in childhood, and in acral sites, but should not be abundant

o *Pagetoid – single or nested melanocytes located above the basal layer of the epidermis*

   Presence implies loss of connection to basement membrane (through either trauma or deranged cellular substructure)

o Maturation in dermis (Fig. 1.5)

   Nevus cells become smaller and darker

   – Abundant cytoplasm and vesicular nuclei in papillary dermis
   – Minimal cytoplasm, small, dark nuclei at base

   Nests become smaller and eventuate in single melanocytes traversing between dermal collagen bundles
   Orderly maturation sequence is the rule – absence raises possibility of melanoma

o Dermal mitoses rare – should never be at base of lesion

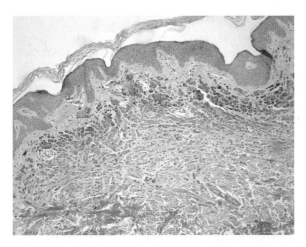

Fig. 1.5 Maturation is a feature of benign melanocytic proliferations. The melanocytes become smaller and darker and the nests become smaller and more widely dispersed with progressive descent into the dermis. Pigmentation also tends to diminish with progressive descent. Original magnification ×100

- Congenital melanocytic nevus
  - Clinical
    - Present in about 1% of newborns
    - Often larger than acquired nevi
    - May be hair-bearing
    - So-called giant congenital nevi (>20 cm) often have a bathing suit distribution
    - Incidence of developing melanoma

      Minimally increased in small congenital nevi
      May be as much as 10% in "giant" nevi

  - Histologic (Figs. 1.6 and 1.7)
    - Can be junctional, compound, or intradermal
    - Abundant single melanocytes within epidermis in some congenital nevi in children
    - Nevus nests extend into lower third of reticular dermis or into subcutis

- o   Nevus nests track down appendages
- o   Nevus nests often have a "superficial perivascular dermatitis" appearance at low magnification

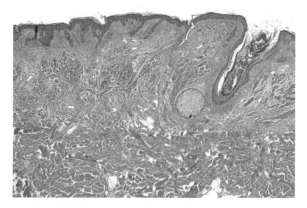

Fig. 1.6 Congenital nevi are characterized by dense clusters of melanocytes that fill the superficial dermis and extend into the deeper reticular dermis. Original magnification ×40

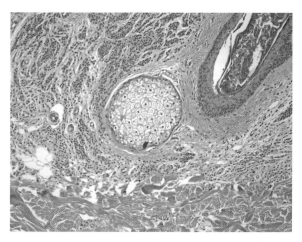

Fig. 1.7 Congenital nevi demonstrate extension of melanocytes around the cutaneous appendages. Original magnification ×100

- Scattered Pagetoid cells may be present in the central portion of congenital nevi, especially during the first year of life
- Pseudovascular spaces are often present and are due to dyscohesion of melanocytes within dermal nests (Fig. 1.8)
- Neurotization is commonly seen and is believed to be part of the maturation process (Fig. 1.9)

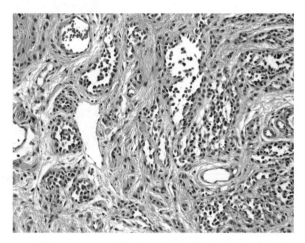

Fig. 1.8 Congenital nevi often demonstrate pseudovascular spaces in the reticular dermis. Original magnification ×200

- Halo nevus

  - Clinical

    - Occurs most commonly on the back and chest of teenagers
    - Central area of pigmentation with circumferential areas of depigmentation
    - Areas of depigmentation progressively expand while pigmented centers shrink
    - Multiple halo nevi (especially in adults) associated with metastastic melanoma and vitiligo (rare)

  - Histologic (Figs. 1.10, 1.11, and 1.12)

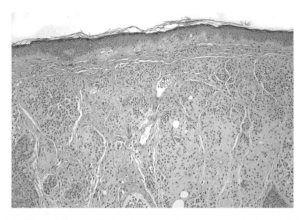

Fig. 1.9 Extensive neurotization is present in many congenital nevi. Original magnification ×100

- o Ordinary appearing nevus with brisk lymphocytic infiltrate
- o Loss of melanocytes within epidermis at lateral edges of lesion (subtle)
- o Melanocytes in central portion of lesion may appear somewhat atypical and rare mitoses may be seen
- o Dyscohesion of melanocytic nests is common in central portion of lesions
- o Maturation difficult to assess because of density of lymphocytic infiltrate

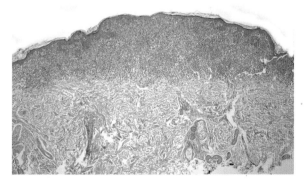

Fig. 1.10 Halo nevi are characterized by a brisk lymphocytic response admixed with melanocytes that can be intradermal or epidermal. Original magnification ×40

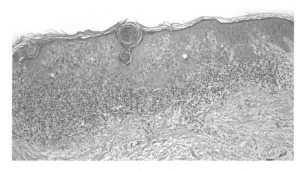

Fig. 1.11 Halo nevi are characterized by nests of melanocytes that may demonstrate reactive atypia and a dense lymphoid infiltrate. Original magnification ×100

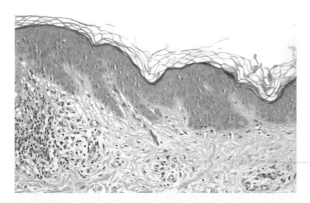

Fig. 1.12 Lateral margins in halo nevi demonstrate a slight lymphoid infiltrate and a loss of intraepidermal melanocytes. Original magnification ×200

- Nevus of special sites (acral, genital, umbilical, breast)
  - Clinical
    - Small, dark nevi arise on palms, soles, genital skin, umbilicus, breasts
    - May appear clinically atypical, but more commonly, concern is over histologic features and not clinical appearance

- Histologic (Figs. 1.13, 1.14, and 1.15)

  o Often increased numbers of single melanocytes relative to numbers of nests in epidermis
  o Pagetoid cells more pronounced than in other types of benign nevi
  o Circumscription less apparent in some cases
  o Intraepidermal melanocytes may appear somewhat atypical – either large, epithelioid cells or markedly hyperchromatic
  o Dermal process is similar to that seen in common acquired nevi

- Combined nevus

  - Histologic (Figs. 1.16 and 1.17)

    o A purely histologic term given to nevi that display more than one type of differentiation, i.e., combined blue and intradermal nevus or combined Spitz and compound nevus

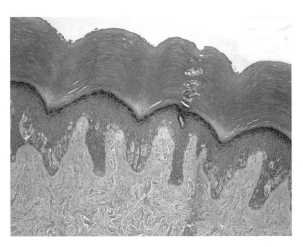

Fig. 1.13 Acral nevi are characterized by increased numbers of single melanocytes within the epidermis with scattered Pagetoid (*upward*) migration. Original magnification ×100

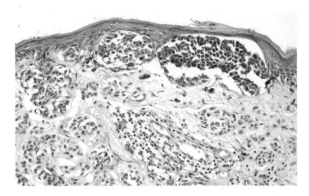

Fig. 1.14 Genital nevi often demonstrate large nests of melanocytes within the epidermis that may become dyscohesive and demonstrate cytologic atypia. Original magnification ×200

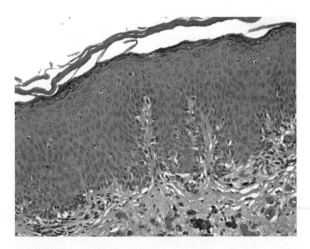

Fig. 1.15 Genital nevi may also be characterized by single melanocytes along the dermal–epidermal junction. Original magnification ×200

- o Of no consequence in terms of prognosis, but important to recognize as distinct from melanoma
- o Diagnosis often is rendered as combined nevus subsequently listing the histologic patterns observed

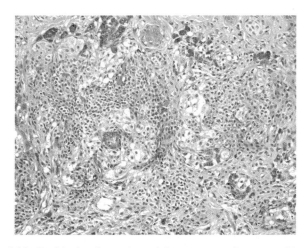

Fig. 1.16 Combined melanocytic nevi demonstrate melanocytes with more than one morphologic form as is seen in this case with smaller cells admixed with a population of larger, more epithelioid, and deeply pigmented cells. Original magnification ×200

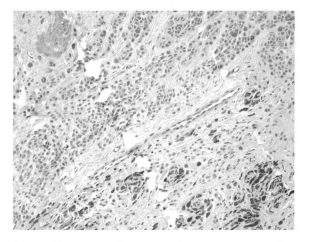

Fig. 1.17 Combined nevi can have many different combinations of cell types including a conventional compound and blue nevus as is seen in this example. Original magnification ×200

Chapter 2
Essential Criteria for Diagnosing Melanoma

- Essential criteria for diagnosing melanoma
  - Major histologic subtypes
    - Helpful to subdivide in order to discuss differing histologic criteria for establishing diagnosis
    - Superficial spreading, nodular, lentigo maligna melanoma, acral lentiginous, mucosal lentiginous
    - No longer thought to be valid as a prognostic indicator (in most cases)
- Superficial spreading melanoma (Figs. 2.1 and 2.2)
  - Most common subtype (50–75%)
  - Histologic features:
    - Intraepidermal features

      Poorly circumscribed melanocytic proliferation
      Asymmetrical
      Pagetoid cells – almost always present in this subtype ("buckshot scatter")
      Dyscohesive melanocytes within nests
      Cytologic atypia – usually epithelioid cell type – large open nuclei and prominent nucleoli; also small cell variant (see below)
      Melanocytes may extend down cutaneous appendages

B.R. Smoller, K.M. Hiatt, *Epidermal Cell Tumors: The Basics*,
DOI 10.1007/978-1-4419-7704-5_2,
© Springer Science+Business Media, LLC 2011

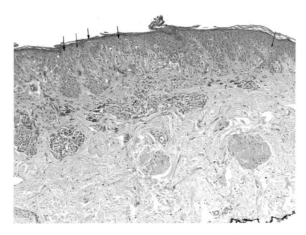

Fig. 2.1 Superficial spreading melanoma is characterized by a poorly circumscribed melanocytic proliferation with numerous Pagetoid cells (*arrows*) and epithelioid cytology

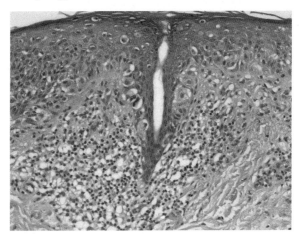

Fig. 2.2 Melanocytes with epithelioid cytology are seen extending down the adnexal epithelium in this case of superficial spreading melanoma

   o Dermal features

      Lack of maturation (see Chapter 1 for definition)
      Mitotic activity in deeper parts of proliferation

Cytologic atypia – usually big, epithelioid cells

Vascular invasion may be present

Perineural invasion may be present, but not as common as in desmoplastic subtype

Host response – often brisk in "radial growth phase" lesions – difficult concept histologically

- Radial growth phase

  o Characteristic of superficial spreading melanoma, absent in nodular melanoma
  o Defined as microinvasion into dermis with nests and single cells that resemble intraepidermal melanoma cells
  o Dermal nests of melanoma cells are smaller than those in epidermis
  o Mitoses are not identified
  o Metastasis rare at this stage

- Vertical growth phase

  o Dermal cells and nests may be larger than those in epidermis
  o Dermal mitoses may be present
  o All melanomas that are levels III or IV (see below) and some that are level II may be in vertical growth phase
  o Vertical growth phase has the potential to metastasize
  o *However, the distinction between radial and vertical growth phase can be dependent on specimen processing as well as reader interpretation and difficult to apply*
  o Attempts have been made to look at proliferative index using Ki-67 and MIB-1 immunohistochemical stains

    Most nodular melanomas have >10% of cells expressing proliferation markers (Fig. 2.3)

    Immunostaining for mitotic activity is rapidly becoming standard practice in difficult melanocytic lesions

- Nodular melanoma

  - Accounts for 15–35% of all melanomas
  - Histologic features (Figs. 2.4 and 2.5):

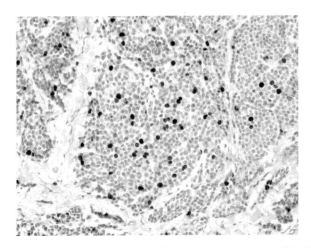

Fig. 2.3 The proliferative index of this melanoma is assessed with Ki-67 immunohistochemical staining. This melanoma, as in most, shows >10% of tumor cells expressing this marker

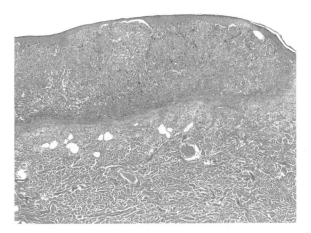

Fig. 2.4 Nodular melanomas show relative circumscription compared to the superficial spreading subtype

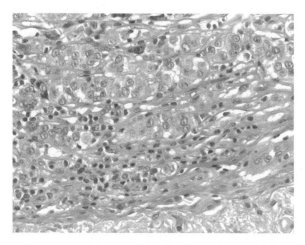

Fig. 2.5 The dermal component of nodular melanomas is composed of cells that fail to mature as seen in the deep component of this melanoma. Note that these melanocytes have large nuclei, open chromatin pattern, and prominent nucleoli at the base of the infiltrate

- Similar to superficial spreading melanoma, but less prominent epidermal changes
- Poor circumscription is not a feature (usually well-circumscribed and often symmetrical at scanning magnification)
- No "radial growth phase" – important biologically but often difficult to assess histologically (see above section)
- Dermal changes identical to superficial spreading melanoma – usually big, epithelioid cell type; also a small cell variant
- Variable host response
- Brisk mitotic rate in many cases
- Marked pleomorphism in majority of cases

• Lentigo maligna melanoma (Figs. 2.6 and 2.7)

– Accounts for 5–15% of all melanomas
– Definitions:

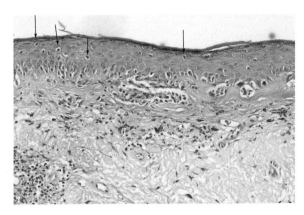

Fig. 2.6 This lentigo maligna shows the characteristic atrophic epidermis with a proliferation of melanocytes along the basilar layer. As is characteristic, these melanocytes show hyperchromatic nuclei. Pagetoid extension is noted (*arrows*). The dermis shows extensive solar elastosis

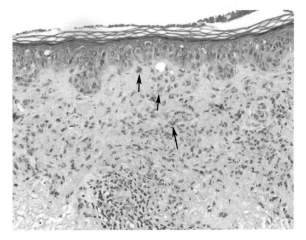

Fig. 2.7 In this example, lentigo maligna melanoma is composed of less characteristic plump melanocytes. The epidermis is atrophic and extensive solar elastosis is noted. Note the melanocytes with similar epithelioid morphology extending into the superficial dermis (*arrows*)

- o Lentigo maligna is a subtype of melanoma in situ occurring in the setting of extensively sun-damaged skin
- o Lentigo maligna melanoma is the same histologic subtype that has evolved to invade the underlying dermis

- – Histologic features:

  - o Epidermal features

    Atrophic epidermis with flattened rete ridges
    Runs of single, confluent melanocytes along basal layer
    Hyperchromatic melanocytes with contracted cytoplasm (leaving apparent halo) is the most common cytology of the melanocytes: this is very different than the melanocytes in superficial spreading/nodular types
    Rare Pagetoid extension. May occur later in course
    Tendency for intraepidermal nesting late in course
    Runs of melanocytes tracking down appendages
    "Starburst" giant cells (multinucleated melanocytes in basal layer – occasional feature)
    Haphazard distribution of melanocytes along basal layer

  - o Dermal features

    Takes 10–50 years before invasion occurs according to some experts
    Marked solar elastosis
    Hyperchromatic, spindle-shaped (usually) melanocytes in fascicles in dermis – often remarkably uniform in appearance
    Prominent host response
    Perineural invasion
    Mitotic activity
    Lack of maturation
    Stromal response not uncommon (fibrotic, desmoplastic, even myxoid)

- – Assessing dermal microinvasion (Fig. 2.8):

  - o Host inflammatory response (often lichenoid)
  - o Fibrosis

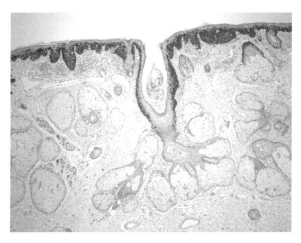

Fig. 2.8 Immunohistochemical staining can be helpful in delimiting the extent of a melanocytic proliferation. But caution is advised in using it to establish microinvasion as melanophages and benign pre-existing components can also express these markers

- o Melanophage accumulation
- o Neovascularization
- o Immunostains are not helpful to identify microinvasion by scattered cells:

  S100 may stain non-melanocytes, i.e., dermal dendritic cells

  HMB-45/MART-1 may stain benign nevus cells and may miss spindle-shaped cells

  Unclear prognostic significance to find one to two cells only with immunostains

- Acral lentiginous melanoma (Figs. 2.9, 2.10, and 2.11)

  - Accounts for 5–10% of all melanomas
  - Histologic features:

    - o Epithelial features

      Site specific

      Increased numbers of single, spindle-shaped melanocytes in lentiginous growth pattern

      Acanthotic epidermis with elongated rete ridges

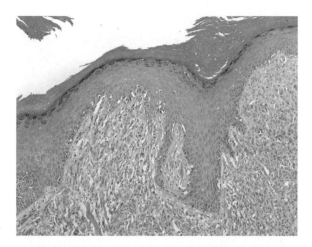

Fig. 2.9   Increased single melanocytes along the basilar layer of an acanthotic epidermis are characteristic of acral lentiginous melanomas

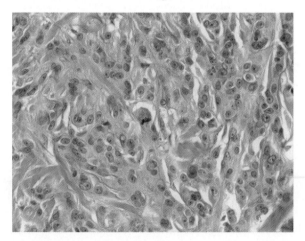

Fig. 2.10   As in other subtypes of melanoma, the dermal component of acral lentiginous melanoma shows mitoses, prominent nucleoli, pleomorphism, and poor maturation characterized by open nuclei

      Poor circumscription
      Pagetoid cells – may have "buckshot" scatter, but not as
         prominent as in superficial spreading melanoma
      Dyscohesion of nests (when present)

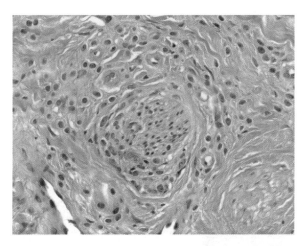

Fig. 2.11 Perineural involvement is commonly seen in acral lentiginous melanoma

  o Dermal/mucosal features

    Spindle-shaped cells coursing in fascicles
    Less commonly described are giant cells, nevoid cells, and
      clear cells in dermis
    Cytologic atypia – hyperchromasia, pleomorphism
    Lack of maturation
    Mitotic activity
    Tendency for extension down adnexal structures
    Perineural and perivascular invasion not uncommon in
      these lesions

- Mucosal lentiginous melanoma (Fig. 2.12)

  – Accounts for a very small percentage of all melanomas
  – Occurs in

    o mouth, nasal mucosa, and esophagus – 55%
    o vulva – 18%
    o anal canal – 24%
    o penis – 3%

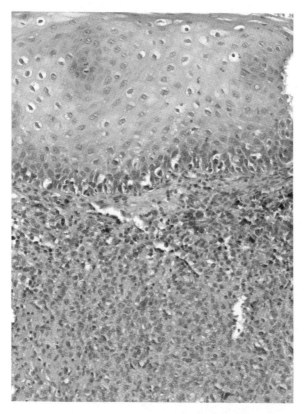

Fig. 2.12 Melanoma arising on mucosal surfaces, such as this rectal melanoma, can show a single cell melanocytic proliferation similar to acral lentiginous melanoma

- Histologic features:

  ○ Most patients present with early dermal invasion
  ○ 50% resemble superficial spreading melanoma, 15% acral lentiginous pattern, mixed pattern in remainder
  ○ Pagetoid spread in epithelium correlates with invasion into dermis
  ○ Lentiginous growth pattern often with spindle-shaped dermal cells and may be associated with desmoplastic stromal response

- o Confluent lentiginous pattern within mucosa associated with angulated nuclei and often dense pigmentation and many dendritic cells

- – Melanoma in situ (synonyms: Hutchinson's melanotic freckle, active junctional nevus, intraepithelial melanocytic neoplasia)

  - o Definition: presence of malignant cells confined to the epidermis without violating the basement membrane
  - o Analogous to ductular carcinoma in situ of the breast or "CIN3" of the cervix
  - o Histologic criteria

    Identical to those for melanoma but changes restricted to the epidermis
    Poor symmetry and circumscription
    Single melanocytes predominate over nests
    Pagetoid extension
    Atypical melanocytes
    Dyscohesion

- Prognostic factors for melanoma

  - – Breslow thickness
  - – Clark's level, for melanoma <1 mm
  - – Ulceration
  - – Mitotic rate/mitotic index
  - – Satellitosis
  - – Vascular invasion
  - – Site
  - – Host response
  - – Regression
  - – Gender

- Breslow thickness

  - – Definition:

    - o Measurement from the most superficial nucleated cell in epidermis (in the granular layer, if present) to the deepest dermal cell that is clearly identifiable as a melanoma cell

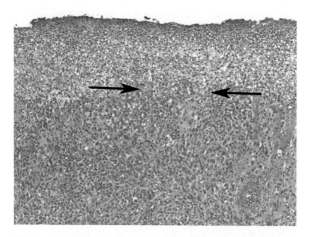

Fig. 2.13 For ulcerated melanomas, the Breslow depth begins at the base of the ulcer (*arrows*), not including the overlying fibrinous material

- o Synonymous with tumor thickness
- o Single most important prognostic feature – this is the primary determinant of T staging
- – Breslow measurement (Figs. 2.13, 2.14, and 2.15)
  - o Caveats:
    Do not measure cells entrapped in adventitial collagen surrounding cutaneous appendages. If this is the only site of invasion, then measure from innermost layer of outer root sheath to melanoma cell
    Do not include underlying associated benign nevi in depth measurement
    In situ melanomas do not have a Breslow thickness
    Ulcerated lesions are measured from the base of the ulcer and a comment as to presence of ulceration must be included
    If a cleft is present, do not include this space in the measurement (subtract cleft space from total measurement)

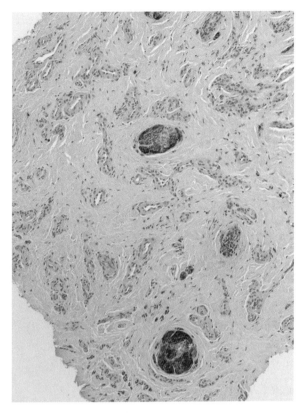

Fig. 2.14 Extensive tracking of the melanoma along eccrine ducts is commonly seen in acral melanomas. S-100 immunohistochemical staining in this case highlights the tracking

- Clark's level
  - Level of the skin into which the melanoma cells most deeply extend:
    - I - intraepidermal (in situ)
    - II - tumor cells extend into papillary dermis
    - III - tumor cells fill and expand the papillary dermis
    - IV - tumor cells extend into reticular dermis
    - V - tumor cells extend into subcutaneous fat

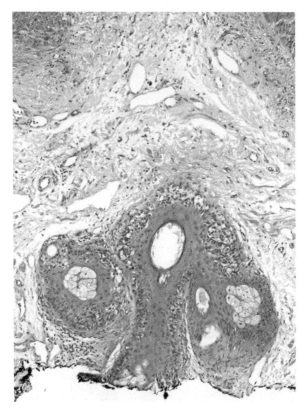

Fig. 2.15 Some melanomas show significant tracking along adnexal structures, including to the base of the specimen, as in this case. This is not to be interpreted as invasion

- Straightforward to identify levels I, IV, V in most cases
  - Often difficult to separate level II from level III. Is it simply filling or filling and expanding the papillary dermis?
- Also can be difficult separate level II from level IV. There are cells not filling and expanding, but just percolating into the papillary dermis and there are rare cells beneath the superficial vascular plexus, i.e., level II or level IV?

- Breslow vs. Clark vs. both

  - Breslow thickness provides much more prognostic information and is much more reproducible
  - On areas of body with extreme skin thicknesses (i.e., eyelids, palms), Clark's level can provide additional prognostic information
  - Clark levels have no prognostic significance for tumors >1 mm thick

- Ulceration

  - The 2002 American Joint Committee on Cancer (AJCC) staging system added ulceration as a major staging criterion
  - Presence of ulceration upstages the melanoma

- Satellitosis

  - Microsatellites are discrete, noncontiguous nests of melanocytes, clearly separated from the main body of the tumor by normal reticular dermal collagen or subcutaneous fat
  - Microsatellites are closely tied to other markers of melanoma behavior – they do appear to predict locoregional relapse
  - They do not determine risk for distant metastases or overall survival
  - Patients with microsatellite lesions have a significantly decreased disease-free survival

- Tumor mitotic rate (Fig. 2.16)

  - Debatable whether tumor ulceration or mitotic index should be considered second in prognostic importance, next to tumor thickness
  - Total number of mitoses/mm^2 in the invasive component with the highest mitotic rate ("mitotic hot spot") provides a more consistent guideline than mitoses/high power field (hpf) or number of mitoses in 10 hpf
  - Tumor mitotic rate (TMR) = 0: better survival than those with TMR = 1
  - TMR is a significant independent prognostic factor, staged by 0, 1–4, 5–10 and $\geq$11 mitoses/mm^2

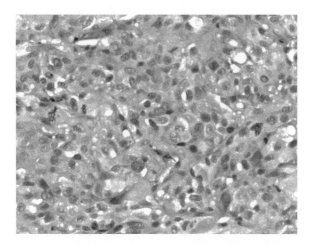

Fig. 2.16 In melanoma, the tumor mitotic rate is determined by finding the most proliferative area, "the hot spot," and determining the number of mitoses/mm^2 on H&E sections

- Vascular involvement
    - Significant increase in the risk of relapse and death when there is vascular invasion with tumor cells in blood or lymphatic vessels *or* uncertain invasion with tumor cells immediately adjacent to endothelium
- Site
    - Some studies show anatomical site to have prognostic significance
    - High-risk sites (BANS acronym):
        - *B*ack
        - Posterior *a*rm
        - *N*eck
        - *S*calp
    - Typically less visible body sites present with thicker tumors – may account for the worse prognosis at these sites

- Lymphocytic infiltrate

  - Early studies showed a "brisk" lymphocytic infiltrate was a favorable feature
  - Presence of "tumor infiltrating lymphocytes" considered a good prognosis in some studies
  - High ratio of the width of the lymphocytic infiltrate compared to the width of the tumor compares with a favorable outcome
  - Significance of lymphocytic infiltrate still controversial

- Regression (Fig. 2.17)

  - Partial regression is not uncommon, found in up to one-third of melanomas
  - More common in thin melanomas
  - May predict a higher risk of metastasis and decreased survival
  - Some studies show no association between regression and metastasis

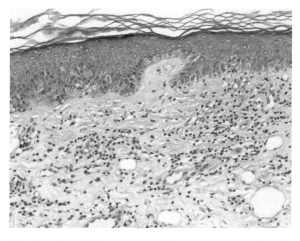

Fig. 2.17 The dermal inflammatory infiltrate, vascular proliferation, and melanophages in a wispy collagenous stroma characterize regression in this example. The depth of the melanoma is not determined by these features, but rather by the adjacent invasive component

- – Some authors advocate including thickness of regression in reports to add additional prognostic information; this is controversial
- Gender
  - – Male gender is associated with a greater incidence of unfavorable primary tumor characteristics
  - – Men with melanoma have an overall lower survival rate than women with melanoma
- Growth patterns
  - – Some evidence suggests that lentigo maligna melanoma, acral lentiginous melanoma, and desmoplastic melanoma may have differing etiology and natural history
    - o lentigo maligna melanoma may have a more favorable prognosis
    - o acral lentiginous melanoma may have a less favorable prognosis
  - – Nonetheless, the same staging criteria should be used for all growth patterns
- Summary
  - – Pathology report must include the features listed in Table 2.1

Table 2.1   Melanoma pathology report

Breslow thickness
Clark's level for T1 tumors (<1 mm thick)
Presence or absence of ulceration
Presence or absence of satellitosis
Host lymphocytic response: brisk vs. non-brisk
Mitoses (#/mm^2)
Involvement of margins
Number of lymph nodes involved (microscopic or macroscopic involvement)
Presence and extent or absence of regression

Chapter 3
Histologic Mimics of Malignant Melanoma

- Melanocytic lesions with some, but not all, of the features of melanoma (Table 3.1)
- Dysplastic nevus (Clark's nevus or atypical nevus)
    - Definition: pigmented lesion with some clinical *and* histologic features of melanoma but with still undetermined biologic behavior
    - Sporadic lesions seen in 1–15% of Caucasian Americans (most series)
    - Relative risk for developing melanoma about 7% (cumulative lifetime risk about 6%)
    - Type D2 dysplastic nevus syndrome (dysplastic nevi on a person with multiple relatives with melanoma and dysplastic nevi) – 20,000–30,000 such patients in USA, cumulative lifetime risk of melanoma approaches 100%
    - Clinical features:
        ○ Usually >0.5 cm in diameter
        ○ Irregular and indistinct margins
        ○ Variegated pigmentation
    - Histologic features:
    - Architectural features (Figs. 3.1, 3.2, 3.3, and 3.4)
        ○ Extension of junctional component of nevus beyond dermal component, "shouldering"
        ○ Anastamosing nests of horizontally oriented melanocytes, "bridging"

B.R. Smoller, K.M. Hiatt, *Epidermal Cell Tumors: The Basics*,
DOI 10.1007/978-1-4419-7704-5_3,
© Springer Science+Business Media, LLC 2011

Table 3.1   Histologic mimics of malignant melanoma

Dysplastic (atypical) nevus
Spindle and epithelioid cell (Spitz) nevus
Pigmented spindle cell nevus
Cellular blue nevus
Deep penetrating nevus
Balloon cell nevus
Acral nevus (nevus of special sites)
Recurrent nevus

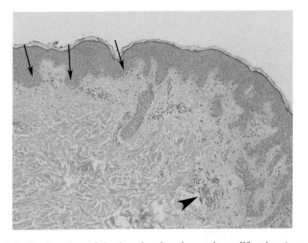

Fig. 3.1 Continuation of the junctional melanocytic proliferation (*arrows*) beyond the dermal component (*arrow head*) is a feature of dysplasia often referred to as "shouldering"

- o Irregular distribution of junctional nests along rete ridges
- o Lentiginous basilar melanocytic hyperplasia (increased numbers of single melanocytes present along elongated rete ridges)
- o Lamellar fibroplasias, concentric eosinophilic fibroplasia
- o Melanophages and lymphocytic infiltrate
- – Cytologic features
  - o Enlarged melanocytes with increased cytoplasm

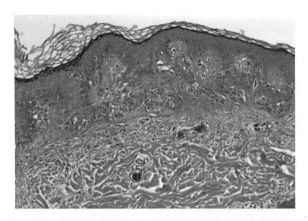

Fig. 3.2 Anastomosing nests of melanocytes, a feature of dysplasia, is seen in this junctional melanocytic nevus

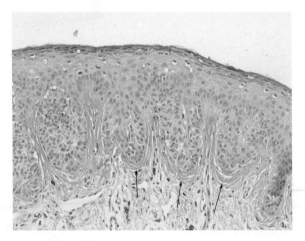

Fig. 3.3 Lamellar fibroplasia, a feature of dysplasia, is represented by eosinophilic bands (*arrows*) in the papillary dermis running parallel to the basilar epithelium

- o Enlarged nuclei and open chromatin pattern
- o Presence of nucleoli within epidermal melanocytes (variable)

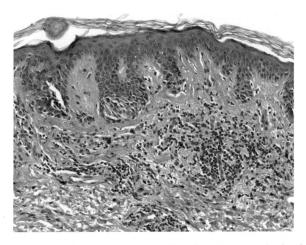

Fig. 3.4 A lymphocytic infiltrate along with melanophages are the dysplastic features seen in this compound nevus

- – Clinical inter-observer reproducibility in making the diagnosis of dysplastic nevus – estimated at 85%
- – Histologic inter-observer reproducibility in making the diagnosis of dysplastic nevus – estimated at 84%
- – Clinicopathologic correlation – 75%
- – Grading degree of dysplasia – very controversial due to lack of complete consensus on criteria and significance of observations
- Spindle and epithelioid cell (Spitz) nevus (Fig. 3.5)
  - – Clinical features
    - ○ >50% occur in patients <20 years of age
    - ○ Often appears as red- or skin-colored papules
    - ○ Melanin not readily apparent in most cases (clinical differential diagnosis usually includes vascular lesion vs. juvenile xanthogranuloma)
    - ○ Rapid onset
    - ○ Any body site, but common on face

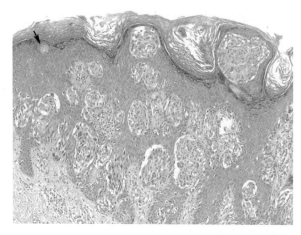

Fig. 3.5 Spitz nevi are composed of melanocytes that have both spindled and epithelioid morphology. Clefting over top of the junctional nests, as seen here, is also characteristic as are eosinophilic epidermal globules (*arrow*) called Kamino bodies

- Histologic features
  - Sharply circumscribed
  - Large nests of melanocytes (vertically oriented) along the dermal–epidermal junction
  - Scattered Pagetoid cells (especially in center of lesions)
  - Clefting around (but not within) nests of melanocytes
  - Frequent epidermal hyperplasia
  - Eosinophilic globules (Kamino bodies) often present
  - Large cells with abundant eosinophilic cytoplasm, vesicular nuclei with prominent nucleoli
  - Dermal maturation with progressive descent must be present
  - Occasional dermal mitoses present, but should not be atypical nor located at base of lesion
- Pigmented spindle cell nevus
  - Clinical features
    - 2:1 female:male ratio

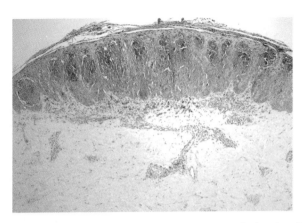

Fig. 3.6 Pigmented spindle cell nevi are well-circumscribed and typically composed of large nests of heavily pigmented as in this one. The acanthotic epidermis seen here is also characteristic

- o 2.5–56 years old, mean 25.3
- o 67% on extremities
- o 33% on trunk
- o 1.6–6.0 mm diameter (2.8 mm avg.)
- o Distinct margins
- o Usually present for only 6–10 months
- o Dark brown-black

- − Histologic features (Fig. 3.6)

  - o Sharp lateral demarcation
  - o Large, discrete nests of junctional melanocytes
  - o Epidermal hyperplasia
  - o 36% junctional nests only, 64% compound nevi
  - o 75% entirely spindle-shaped melanocytes
  - o 25% mixed spindle and epithelioid morphologies
  - o 25% with sparse Pagetoid cells in central portion of lesion
  - o Rare mitoses (none atypical) – should not be at base of dermal component
  - o Uniform nuclear appearance throughout lesion

- 50% with extension down eccrine ducts
- Occasional nucleoli in melanocytes
- 50% with lymphocytic response
- Papillary dermal fibrosis uncommon (in contrast to dysplastic or atypical nevus)

- Cellular blue nevus
  - Clinical features
    - 67% occur in patients less than 40 years old, but range 6–85 years (mean 30)
    - May be slight female predominance
    - 70% in Caucasians
    - Described in prostate, cervix, vaginal, lung, orbit, spermatic cord
    - Sacrococcygeal site most common, acral and scalp also common
    - Most lesions 0.5–1.0 cm, as large as 4.0 cm reported
    - Blue-black dermal nodules without change
    - No epidermal surface changes
    - Uniform color throughout
  - Histologic features (Figs. 3.7, 3.8, and 3.9)
    - Superficial to mid-dermal, may extend into subcutis
    - Intermingled oval-plump, often amelanotic cells with densely pigmented dendritic cells
    - Sclerosis common
    - Mitoses rare (<1/hpf)
    - Can see intermixed neuroid structures
    - Occasional nucleoli
    - Occasional multinucleated cells
    - Overlying junctional cells unusual
    - Atypical cellular blue nevi have increased nuclear:cytoplasmic ratios, increased mitoses, and increased cellularity
    - *Zonal necrosis should not be present – it represents a feature of malignant transformation in these lesions*

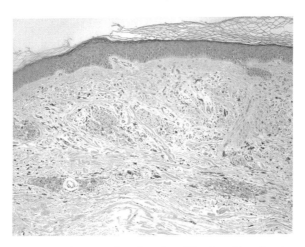

Fig. 3.7 Cellular blue nevus is a dermal proliferation of heavily pigmented spindle cells characteristic of blue nevi, admixed with clusters of oval cells with variable pigmentation. The lack of a junctional component is typical

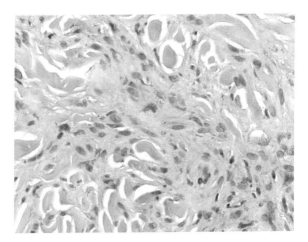

Fig. 3.8 The less pigmented oval cells of a cellular blue nevus have variable pigmentation, larger nuclei, and may have nucleoli. Mitoses, if seen, should be rare

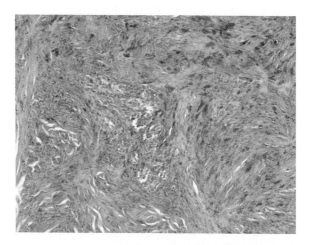

Fig. 3.9 Cellular blue nevi may be densely cellular, as in this one, and may be large, extending to the subcutaneous tissue

- Deep penetrating nevus (plexiform spindle cell nevus)

  - Clinical features

    o Blue-black nodule or papule
    o Often occurs on face and upper trunk
    o Thought (by some) to be variant of a congenital nevus
    o Most common in young adults

  - Histologic features (Figs. 3.10 and 3.11)

    o Minimal or no junctional component
    o Dermal infiltrate with "dumb bell" configuration at base
    o Melanocytic proliferation tracks around hair follicles into deep dermis/subcutaneous fat
    o Nests of ovoid melanocytes with minimal pigment
    o Abundant, heavily pigment-laden melanophages
    o Striking resemblance to blue nevus in some cases and cellular blue nevus in others – differentiated by "dumbbell" configuration of growth pattern
    o Rare mitoses may be present
    o Cytologic atypia sometimes present (ancient change?) but inconspicuous nucleoli

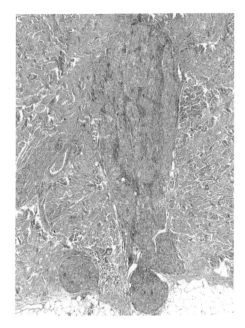

Fig. 3.10 Deep penetrating nevi may extend, with a bulbous or pushing front, along hair follicles, into the subcutaneous tissue

- o No necrosis
- o Spindle-shaped cells predominate over epithelioid ones
- o Maturation in areas away from perifollicular adventitial collagen
- o Nests may infiltrate nerves and arrector pili

- Balloon cell nevus

  - Clinical features

    - o Not specific
    - o May show pigment irregularities which resemble melanoma on clinical evaluation

  - Histologic features (Figs. 3.12 and 3.13)

    - o Partial balloon cell transformation in nevi or melanomas not uncommon, but purely balloon cell process very rare

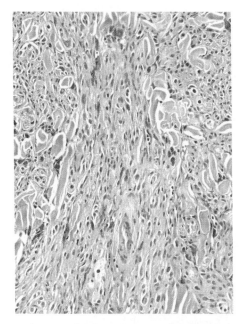

Fig. 3.11 The fascicular growth of deep penetrating nevi, with variable pigmentation, may resemble cellular blue nevus. Mild nuclear atypia may be seen, but mitoses are rare

- o Architectural pattern is that of benign nevus:
- o regularly nested, sharply circumscribed, no Pagetoid cells, good dermal maturation

- – Confusing cytology

  - o Cells are very large, with abundant dusty cytoplasm
  - o Nuclei may be slightly vesicular
  - o Nucleoli inconspicuous

- • Recurrent nevus

  - – Clinical features

    - o New area of pigmentation at site of previously excised (or traumatized) pigmented lesion

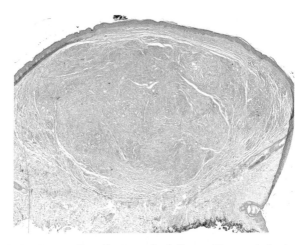

Fig. 3.12 The overall architecture of a balloon cell nevus is benign with circumscription and maturation

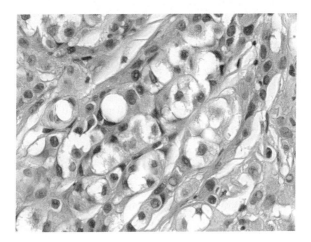

Fig. 3.13 On close inspection, balloon cell nevi have cells with abundant vesicular cytoplasm. Nuclei are slightly larger than surrounding conventional melanocytic cells, which are typically interspersed among those cells with balloon cell change, as in this image

Table 3.2 Differential diagnosis of Pagetoid melanocytes

Melanoma
Spindle and epithelioid cell (Spitz) nevus
Acral nevus (nevus of special sites)
Congenital nevus (especially in infants)
Recurrent nevus
Excoriated nevus

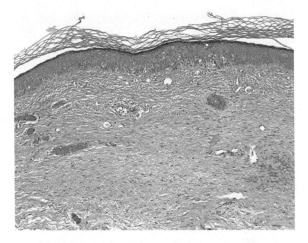

Fig. 3.14 Recurrent nevi are characterized by the sometimes exuberant single melanocytic cell proliferation within the epidermis. The proliferation is limited to the epidermis directly overlying the dermal fibrosis of the previous procedure

  o Often clinically irregular in appearance and potentially
    concerning without history of prior trauma at site
  o Scarring may resemble area of regression

– Histologic features (Figs. 3.14 and 3.15)

  o Nests and single melanocytes immediately overlying der-
    mal scar – irregularly distributed
  o No extension beyond scar

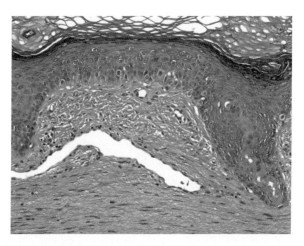

Fig. 3.15 Recurrent nevi are composed predominantly of single melanocytes with rare nests. The melanocytes often have cytologic atypia as in these epithelioid melanocytes

- o Pagetoid cells present but not usually abundant or full thickness (Table 3.2)
- o Dyscohesion frequent
- o Cytologic atypia increased
- o May be residual dermal component surrounding scar

Chapter 4
Epidermal Neoplasms

- Benign keratinocytic lesions
  - Epidermal nevus
  - Prurigo nodularis
  - Granuloma fissuratum
  - Seborrheic keratoses
  - Inverted follicular keratoses
  - Lichenoid keratosis

- Premalignant keratinocytic lesions
  - Actinic keratoses

- Malignant keratinocytic lesions
  - Squamous cell carcinoma
    - Keratoacanthoma type
  - Basal cell carcinoma

- Epidermal nevus
  - Clinical
    - Typically in children
    - Verrucoid plaque on neck, trunk, or extremities
    - Ovoid or linear
    - Tan to brown colored

B.R. Smoller, K.M. Hiatt, *Epidermal Cell Tumors: The Basics*,
DOI 10.1007/978-1-4419-7704-5_4,
© Springer Science+Business Media, LLC 2011

- Histology (Fig. 4.1)

  o Papillomatous
  o Flat-topped, broad papillary projections
  o Hyperkeratosis
  o Hypergranulosis with normal keratohyalin clumping
  o Mild increase in basilar pigmentation may be present

- Prurigo nodularis

  - Clinical

    o Well-circumscribed, firm nodule(s)
    o Varied distribution, most prevalent on extensor surface of extremities
    o Associated with intense pruritus
    o Caused by chronic scratching or rubbing

  - Histology (Figs. 4.2 and 4.3)

    o Dome-shaped
    o Acanthotic epidermis with gradual increase in thickness at margins of nodule

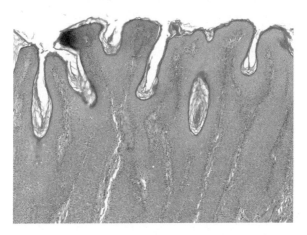

Fig. 4.1 Epidermal nevus on the neck of a 9-year-old girl shows the classic acanthotic epidermis with a papillomatous architecture. Note that the projections have a flat top with mild orthokeratosis

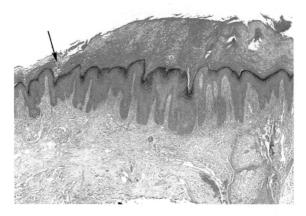

Fig. 4.2 This low-power image of prurigo nodularis shows the dome shape with gradual increase in epidermal acanthosis laterally (*arrow*)

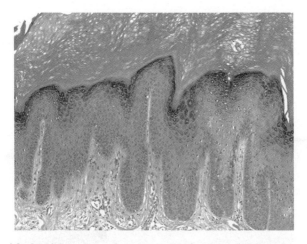

Fig. 4.3 On higher power of prurigo nodularis, notice that there is normal keratohyalin clumping and orthokeratosis

- o Hypergranulosis and hyperkeratosis
- o May have an associated inflammatory infiltrate

- Granuloma fissuratum

  - Clinical

    - o Variation of prurigo nodularis caused by rubbing and pressure
    - o At site of glasses, dentures, or prosthesis
    - o Well-circumscribed, firm nodule(s), with central depression
    - o Painful
    - o May ulcerate

  - Histology (Fig. 4.4)

    - o Dome-shaped
    - o Acanthotic epidermis with irregular, broad, elongated rete
    - o Hypergranulosis
    - o Hyperkeratosis and parakeratosis

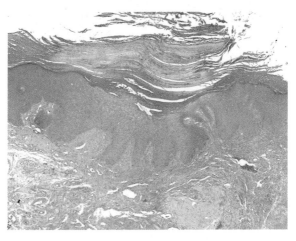

Fig. 4.4 Granuloma fissuratum shows irregular acanthosis with a central depression. Note the lack of a granular cell layer and the overlying parakeratosis at the depression point

- o Central depression, corresponding to clinically noted depression
- o May have epidermal attenuation or ulceration at depression

- Seborrheic keratosis

  - Clinical

    - o Very common in middle aged and elderly
    - o Incidence approximately equal across genders
    - o Arise spontaneously
    - o Round, flat, velvety plaques
    - o May be pigmented
    - o Appear to be "stuck on"
    - o Treatment is unnecessary, except for cosmesis or to rule out malignancy
    - o May become inflamed and irritated
    - o Explosive onset may occur as a *paraneoplastic syndrome*

      Sign of *Leser-Trelat (controversial)*
      Gastric adenocarcinoma, lymphoma, breast cancer, and squamous cell carcinoma of lung
      Thought that transforming growth factor alpha (TGF-α) produced by the tumor may have a role

  - Histology (Figs. 4.5, 4.6, 4.7, 4.8, and 4.9)

    - o Hyperkeratosis without parakeratosis (except may be seen overlying traumatized seborrheic keratoses or in so-called clonal lesions)
    - o Proliferation of homogeneous appearing basaloid keratinocytes
    - o Horn cysts (follicular) lined with cells containing granular cytoplasm and filled with orthokeratotic keratin
    - o Slight underlying papillary dermal fibrosis
    - o Mitoses rare
    - o Trauma to lesion results in increased mitoses, cytologic atypia, spongiosis, and occasional spindle cell transformation of keratinocytes

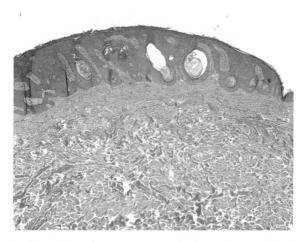

Fig. 4.5 Seborrheic keratosis shows a well-circumscribed proliferation of basaloid cells. As seen here, the base of the lesion is flat. Horn cysts are commonly present and pigmentation may also be noted, as in this lesion

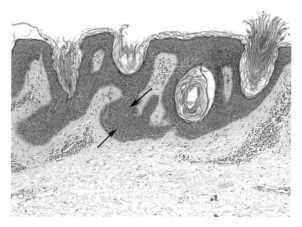

Fig. 4.6 Seborrheic keratoses may have areas of squamatization (*arrow*) which are indicative of trauma or irritation

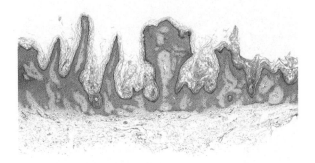

Fig. 4.7 This seborrheic keratosis has a verrucoid architecture and shows the very characteristic flat base

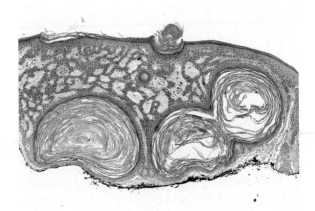

Fig. 4.8 Other less common patterns of seborrheic keratosis include the reticulated pattern shown in this lesion characterized by trabeculae of basaloid cells extending from the epidermis.

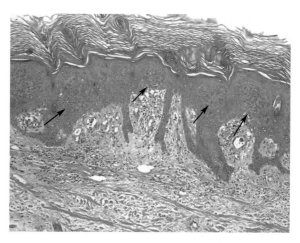

Fig. 4.9 Seborrheic keratosis with the clonal pattern is characterized by intraepidermal nests of cytologically bland keratinocytes (*arrows*)

- Inverted follicular keratoses

    - Clinical

        ○ No unique clinical features
        ○ Resembles seborrheic keratoses
        ○ Most common on the face around the nasal region

    - Histology (Fig. 4.10)

        ○ Cup-shaped invagination filled with keratin
        ○ Keratin is usually orthokeratotic, but may have slight parakeratosis
        ○ Proliferation of basaloid keratinocytes, some of which may become spindle-shaped
        ○ Suprabasilar spongiosis may be present with sparing of basal layer
        ○ Squamous eddies are abundant and most prevalent in the suprabasilar epidermis
        ○ Mitoses increased, but cytologic atypia minimal (and reactive)

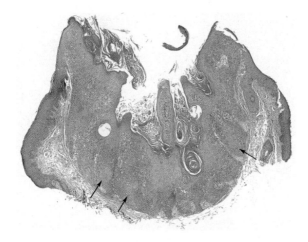

Fig. 4.10 Inverted follicular keratosis shows a cup-shaped invagination of the epidermis filled with orthokeratin. The squamous eddies (*arrows*) most prevalent in the suprabasilar epidermis are also characteristic

- o *Most think inverted follicular keratosis to be a variant of seborrheic keratosis or verruca vulgaris and not a discrete entity*

- Lichenoid keratoses
  - Clinical
    - o Single keratotic lesion occurring most commonly on chest or back
    - o Most common in 5th–7th decades
    - o Clinical differential diagnosis includes basal cell carcinoma and seborrheic keratosis
  - Histology (Figs. 4.11 and 4.12)
    - o Overlying orthokeratosis with focal parakeratosis
    - o Increased thickness to granular layer
    - o Basal keratinocytes with slight cytologic atypia (reactive)
    - o Basal vacuolization may be extensive
    - o Lichenoid or interface (when less intense) inflammatory infiltrate

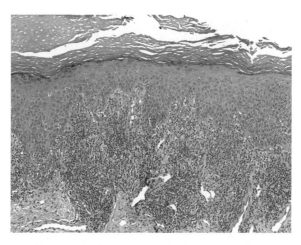

Fig. 4.11 Lichenoid keratosis shows an epidermis with hypergranulosis, over-lying hyperkeratosis and focal parakeratosis. There are scattered dyskeratotic keratinocytes and, in this specimen, a dense lichenoid infiltrate

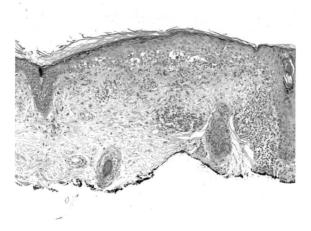

Fig. 4.12 This lichenoid keratosis shows mild hypergranulosis and hyperker-atosis with more extensive interface degeneration. Only a minimal inflamma-tory component is present in this example

- o Inflammation is predominantly lymphocytic
- o Plasma cells and eosinophils may be present in small numbers
- o *Frequently indistinguishable from lichen planus (except by clinical presentation) – see Table* 4.1

Table 4.1 Histologic differences between *Lichen planus* and *Lichenoid keratosis*

Lichen planus	Lichenoid keratosis
Orthokeratosis	Orthokeratosis with occasional parakeratosis (but parakeratosis is not always present)
Inflammation confined to papillary dermis	Papillary dermal inflammation may extend to perivascular regions (but may be confined purely to the papillary dermis)
Eosinophils and plasma cells are very uncommon	Scattered plasma cells and eosinophils are often seen, but there may be a purely lymphocytic infiltrate

- o *Most think lichenoid keratoses to be an inflammatory stage of lentigo simplex, seborrheic keratosis, or verruca*

- Miscellaneous
- Acantholytic acanthoma, dyskeratotic acanthoma

  - Clinical

    - o No specific clinical features
    - o Often believed to be seborrheic keratoses, lichenoid keratoses, or basal cell carcinomas by clinicians

  - Histology (Fig. 4.13)

    - o Small foci of acantholysis or dyskeratoses within epidermis
    - o Cytologic atypia of keratinocytes not present
    - o Hyperkeratosis or parakeratosis often seen overlying foci of change within the epidermis

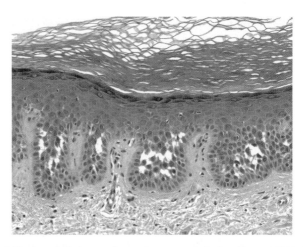

Fig. 4.13 Acantholytic acanthoma shows acantholysis without striking keratinocyte atypia. Overlying hyperkeratosis, as in this lesion, or parakeratosis is usually present

- o Foci could resemble changes seen in Grover's disease, but occur in a single lesion and may be broader than the tiny foci characteristic of Grover's disease
- o Underlying inflammatory response may be present but often absent

- Actinic keratosis
  - Clinical
    - o Ill-defined, scaly plaques
    - o Tan, red, or skin colored
    - o Sun-exposed skin
    - o Excess keratin buildup may cause cutaneous horn (same as in squamous cell carcinoma)
    - o "Pre-cancerous" skin growth – will evolve to fully transformed squamous cell carcinoma in a very small percentage of cases (1–5%) if left untreated

- Histology (Figs. 4.14, 4.15, and 4.16)

  o Parakeratosis, either diffuse or sparing outflow tracts of cutaneous appendages
  o Keratinocyte atypia, usually starting with basal layer
  o Increased nuclear:cytoplasmic ratio and increased cell size
  o Atypia progresses from the basilar layer to the granular cell layer with disease progression (may be thought of as analogous to cervical epithelial CIN I–III)
  o Frequent loss of granular layer (especially underlying zones of parakeratosis)
  o Increased numbers of downward projections (buds) from the surface (appears as if greatly increased numbers of rete ridges)
  o Increased suprabasilar mitotic activity
  o There is underlying solar elastosis, by definition
  o Widely varied degrees of underlying inflammation (from none to lichenoid)
  o Often sparing of cutaneous appendages (even within the epidermal outflow tracts)

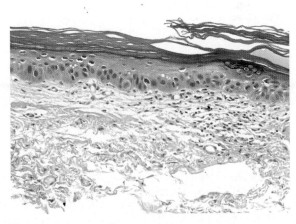

Fig. 4.14 Actinic keratosis is characterized by cytologic atypia in the basilar keratinocytes, overlying hyperkeratosis and solar elastosis

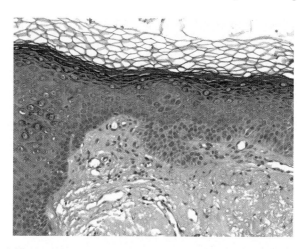

Fig. 4.15 Note the focality of the basilar keratinocyte atypia in this actinic keratosis. The follicular epithelium (*on the left*) is unaffected. Mild hyperkeratosis and abundant solar elastosis are also present

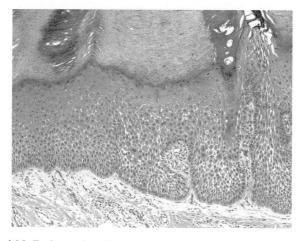

Fig. 4.16 Exuberant hyperkeratosis, resulting in a cutaneous horn, may be present in actinic keratosis. Additionally, acantholysis, as seen in this specimen, may occasionally be present

- Pathophysiology
  - A series of progressively dysplastic changes
  - Related to cumulative sun exposure
  - Unclear what percentage of these lesions progress to malignancy (but a low number often cited as from 1 to 5%)

- Squamous cell carcinoma
  - Clinical
    o Second most common tumor on sun-exposed skin in older people (basal cell carcinoma is most common)
    o Keratotic patch or plaque that is often ulcerated
    o May be erythematous if there is an associated immune response
    o Predisposing factors (collectively, these cause far less squamous cell carcinomas than does chronic sun exposure)

    Industrial carcinogens
    Chronic ulcers
    Draining osteomyelitis
    Old burn scars
    Arsenic ingestion
    Ionizing radiation
    Tobacco chewing
    Ultraviolet light – most common
    Immunosuppression

    - Chemotherapy
    - Organ transplant

    Xeroderma pigmentosa (defective DNA repair)

  - Histology (Figs. 4.17, 4.18, 4.19, and 4.20)
    o Keratinocytic atypia
    o Increased suprabasilar mitoses
    o Often increased numbers of dying keratinocytes
    o In situ stage defined as full-thickness intraepidermal atypia (on the other end of the spectrum from actinic keratoses)

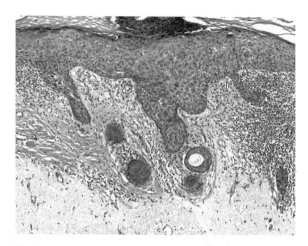

Fig. 4.17 Squamous cell carcinoma shows full-thickness keratinocyte atypia without extension into the dermis. A variable host immune response is present in the dermis that typically has solar elastosis

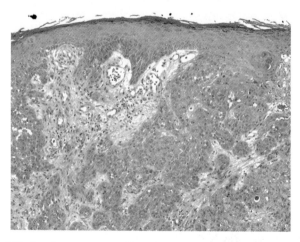

Fig. 4.18 Invasive squamous cell carcinoma showing extension of atypical keratinizing cells throughout the dermis

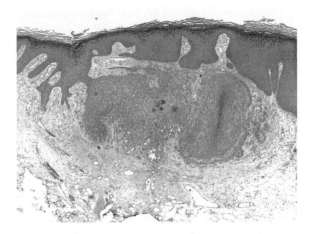

Fig. 4.19 As in this example, invasive squamous cell carcinoma may arise in the skin that does not show full-thickness epidermal atypia

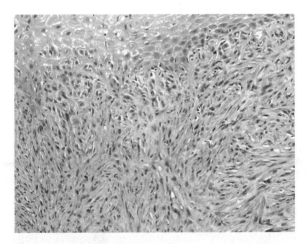

Fig. 4.20 In spindled squamous cell carcinoma, or sarcomatoid squamous cell carcinoma, it may be difficult to ascertain the origin of the lesion from the overlying epidermis. Additionally, these poorly differentiated cells may not express cytokeratin. However, the nuclei will be positive for p63 by immunohistochemistry (see Volume I)

- o Invasion defined as atypical keratinocytes extending through the basement membrane into the underlying dermis
- o Dermal invasion may occur without full-thickness keratinocyte atypia in the overlying epidermis
- o Diffuse parakeratosis frequently present
- o Underlying solar elastosis is present in most cases (related to chronic sunlight exposure) but not seen in squamous cell carcinomas caused by other predisposing factors
- o An associated inflammatory response is highly variable, ranging from diffuse and extensive to virtually none
- o Keratinocytes may have spindle-shaped morphology
- o Acantholysis may be present
- o Perineural and vascular invasion important to note for prognostic reasons
- o Depth of invasion may be important for prognosis (but still controversial)
- o Degree of squamous differentiation (poorly to well-differentiated) does not correlate with overall prognosis

- Pathogenesis

  - Ultraviolet light inhibits Langerhans cell antigen presentation resulting in defective immunosurveillance
  - Ultraviolet light also promotes DNA mutations in keratinocytes leading to malignant transformation through inactivation of p53 tumor suppressor gene

- Keratoacanthoma subtype

  - Clinical

    - o Rapidly developing neoplasm
    - o Clinically and histologically mimics squamous cell carcinoma
    - o Generally >50 years old
    - o Equal incidence in men and women
    - o Sun-exposed skin: ears, nose, cheek, and dorsum of hand
    - o Flesh-colored, dome-shaped nodule

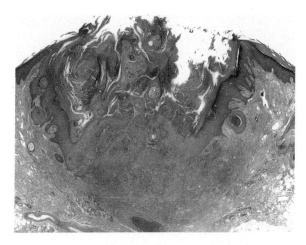

Fig. 4.21 Keratoacanthoma-type squamous cell carcinoma has an invaginated epithelium filled with parakeratotic and orthokeratotic keratin

- o Central keratin-filled plug
- o Spontaneous resolution without treatment in some cases
- o Rapid onset of keratoacanthomas associated with syndromes
- o Multiple keratoacanthomas associated with Muir–Torre syndrome

- Histology (Figs. 4.21 and 4.22)

  - o Cup-shaped invagination with keratin-filled crater
  - o Parakeratosis and orthokeratosis may be present in stratum corneum
  - o Proliferation of large keratinocytes with abundant glassy, pale-staining cytoplasm
  - o Increased mitoses and dying keratinocytes
  - o Cytologic atypia often slight
  - o Dermal invasion often present
  - o Underlying immune response in various stages:

    Marked lymphocytic infiltrate
    Vascular proliferation

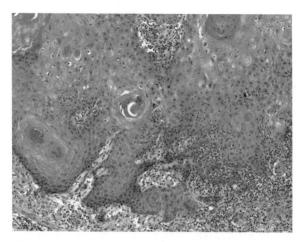

Fig. 4.22 The keratinocytes in keratoacanthoma-type squamous cell carcinoma have abundant eosinophilic cytoplasm, without an elevated nuclear:cytoplasmic ratio. Numerous dying keratinocytes, characterized by darker eosinophilic cytoplasm and smaller hyperchromatic nuclei, may be present

    Increased fibrosis
    Late-stage lesions with flattened epidermal base overlying
       what appears to be a dense dermal scar
  o Perineural invasion described in some cases
 – Pathophysiology
  o Not well-characterized
  o *Very controversial if this is a distinct entity from squa-
     mous cell carcinoma – most authors now consider ker-
     atoacanthoma to be a distinct subtype of squamous cell
     carcinoma, characterized by rapid growth rate and spon-
     taneous involution in some cases if left untreated*

• Basal cell carcinoma
 – Clinical
  o Relatively common

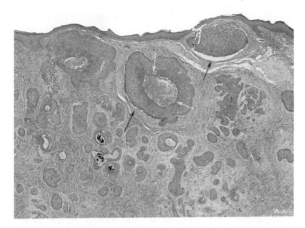

Fig. 4.23 Nodular basal cell carcinoma is the most common and shows nests of basaloid cells in the dermis. Clefting between the nests of basaloid cells and the surrounding stroma (*black arrows*) is characteristic. Central necrosis (*white arrows*) is common in large nests. Calcification and mucin deposition are also commonly seen

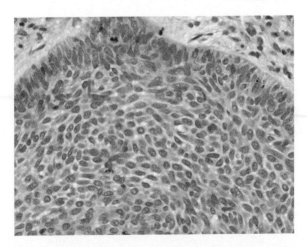

Fig. 4.24 This higher power image of nodular basal cell carcinoma shows the nuclei at the periphery of the nodule aligning next to each other (peripheral palisading). Note also the large nuclei and mitoses

- o Slow growing
- o Rarely metastasize
- o Occurs on sun-exposed skin
- o Pearly papule with telangiectasia
- o Large tumors may ulcerate, so-called rodent ulcers
- o Increased incidence in patients with immunosuppression and in patients with defective DNA repair/replication
- o Associated with long-term chronic sun exposure

- Histology (Figs. 4.23, 4.24, 4.25, 4.26, 4.27, 4.28, and 4.29)

  - o Several morphologic variants with prognostic significance (mainly due to rates of local recurrence)

  Nodular
  Superficial

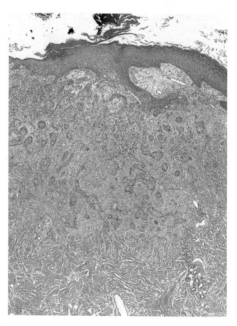

Fig. 4.25 The angulated fingers of basaloid projecting in the deep dermis characterize the infiltrative type of basal cell carcinoma

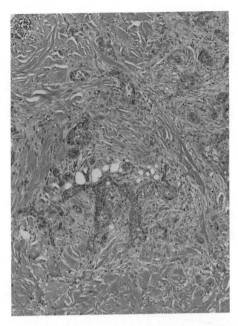

Fig. 4.26 Higher power of infiltrative basal cell carcinoma shows the angulated, slender islands percolating through dermal collagen

   Infiltrative
   Morpheaform
   Micronodular
   Cystic

– All histologic subtypes share some features

   o Nests of basaloid keratinocytes with increased nuclear:-cytoplasmic ratio
   o Peripheral palisade of keratinocytes
   o Increased mitoses
   o Increased numbers of apoptotic cells
   o Myxoid stroma with increased numbers of fibroblasts
   o Cleft artifact not always seen, but helpful when present

– Nodular variant grows as large dermal tumor nodules extending into dermis

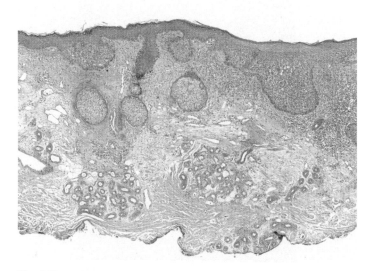

Fig. 4.27 Superficial-type basal cell carcinoma is characterized by basaloid nests of cells with peripheral palisading appearing from multiple origins along the basilar epidermis

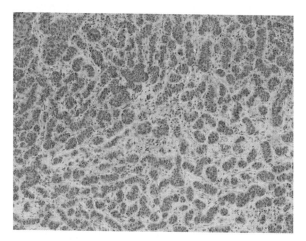

Fig. 4.28 In micronodular basal cell carcinoma, the nests are composed of small aggregates of basaloid cells comprised of only a peripheral layer of cells. Peripheral palisading is often lost in these small aggregates

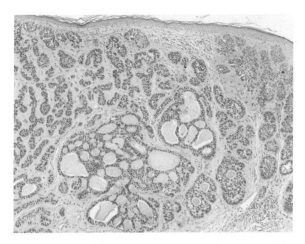

Fig. 4.29 In cystic basal cell carcinoma there is single or multiple cystic spaces within the basaloid nests

- Superficial variant grows down from epidermis, often at several different foci within a single biopsy specimen
- Morpheaform variant has smaller, angulated nests of keratinocytes coursing through abundant myxoid or (less commonly) sclerotic stroma

  o Tends to be more deeply invasive and may extend into muscle or subcutaneous fat

- Micronodular and infiltrative variants have smaller nests of keratinocytes that are either rounded (micronodular) or angulated (infiltrative), coursing through abundant stroma

  o Keratinocyte nests are intermediate in size between nodular variant and morpheaform variant

- Classification of subtypes important for determining biologic behavior

  o Superficial and nodular variants with lowest rate of local recurrence
  o Micronodular and infiltrative variants with intermediate rates of local recurrence

o Morpheaform variant with highest rate of local recurrence

- Extramammary Paget's disease
  - Clinical
    o Most common in anogenital region
    o Can occur in axilla (rare) or many other sites
    o Erythematous, often oozing patch or plaque with slight overlying scale

  - Histologic features (Fig. 4.30)
    o Scattered atypical cells within epidermis with pale-staining cytoplasm
    o Often suprabasilar – rarely clustered
    o Cells present at all levels of epidermis, but often spare the basal layer
    o Cytoplasm may stain with mucicarmine
    o Rare cases with dermal invasion

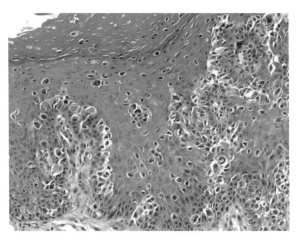

Fig. 4.30 Extramammary Paget shows numerous atypical cells at all levels of the epidermis. These cells are primarily singly dispersed

- Immunostaining

  o Tumor cells express cytokeratin 7
  o Less specifically, also express carcinoembryonic antigen (CEA) and epithelial membrane antigen (EMA), gross cystic fluid protein (GCFP)
  o Histochemical stains are much less specific and probably no longer worth performing to establish this diagnosis

- Pathogenesis

  o Tumors probably arise from apocrine (or less likely eccrine) glands in the skin
  o 20% of cases associated with primary tumors of gastrointestinal or genitourinary tracts. In these cases, tumor cells represent intraepidermal spread of the primary tumor

Chapter 5
Pilosebaceous Neoplasms

- Follicular neoplasms

    - Trichofolliculoma
    - Trichoepithelioma

        o Trichoadenoma
        o Trichoblastoma

    - Pilomatricoma
    - Trichilemmoma
    - Proliferating trichilemmal tumor
    - Fibrofolliculoma
    - Trichodiscoma
    - Tumor of follicular infundibulum

- Trichofolliculoma (TF)

    - Clinical

        o Solitary lesion on face of adults
        o Dome-shaped, skin-colored papule
        o Central port with tuft of hair emerging

    - Histologic

        o Central large cystic space lined with squamous epithelium and filled with keratin and hair fragments (Fig. 5.1)
        o Multiple well-formed hair buds, some with central hairs, surround the central cavity

B.R. Smoller, K.M. Hiatt, *Epidermal Cell Tumors: The Basics*, 75
DOI 10.1007/978-1-4419-7704-5_5,
© Springer Science+Business Media, LLC 2011

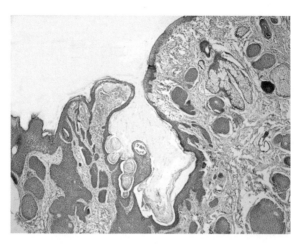

Fig. 5.1 Trichofolliculoma demonstrates a central dell surrounded by basaloid follicular structures. Original magnification ×40

- o May see papillary mesenchymal bodies, other follicular differentiation in buds
- o Follicular buds may appear simply as proliferations of basaloid keratinocytes
- o Can be associated with sebaceous differentiation (sebaceous trichofolliculoma)
- o *Differential diagnosis:*

  Dilated pore of Winer – no surrounding buds
  Pilar sheath acanthoma – trichofolliculoma is more basaloid, pilar sheath acanthoma restricted to upper lip

- Trichoepithelioma
  - Clinical
    - o Single or multiple (autosomal dominant if multiple)
    - o Skin-colored papules, usually on face
    - o Associated with multiple cylindromas (Brooke syndrome)
    - o Best thought of as part of a spectrum with trichoblastoma (least differentiated) and trichoadenoma (most completely differentiated)

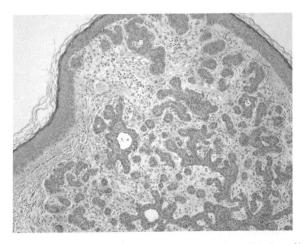

Fig. 5.2 Trichoepithelioma shows a well-circumscribed proliferation of basaloid cells forming islands coursing within fibrous stroma. Original magnification ×100

- Histologic (Fig. 5.2)

  o Well-circumscribed dermal tumor
  o Basaloid cells without significant palisading
  o Central horn cysts filled with keratin
  o Papillary mesenchymal bodies virtually diagnostic (Fig. 5.3)
  o Calcification and foreign body giant cell reaction common
  o No myxoid stroma and no cleft formation (as in basal cell carcinoma)
  o Stroma may be cellular but is more eosinophilic than seen in basal cell carcinoma
  o *Any tumor with "epithelioma" in its name suggests mimic of basal cell epithelioma/carcinoma*

- Desmoplastic type (Figs. 5.4 and 5.5)

  o Abundant desmoplastic stroma
  o Poorly circumscribed
  o Infiltrates into surrounding dermal collagen
  o Differential diagnosis includes

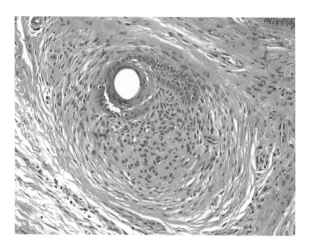

Fig. 5.3 Papillary mesenchymal bodies when present are helpful in distinguishing trichoepitheliomas from basal cell carcinomas. Original magnification ×200

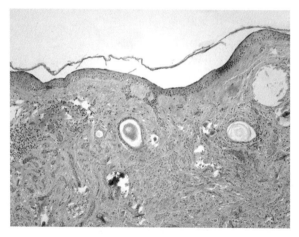

Fig. 5.4 Desmoplastic trichoepithelioma has islands of basaloid cells widely separated by densely fibrotic stroma. Calcification is usually abundant. Original magnification ×100

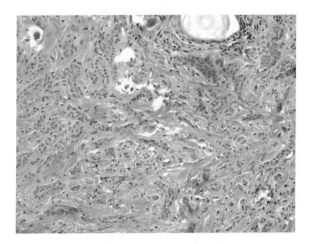

Fig. 5.5 Desmoplastic trichoepithelioma has nuclei that do not overlap and minimal cytologic atypia. Clefting artifact, characteristic of basal cell carcinoma, is not seen. Original magnification ×200

> Morpheic (morpheaform) basal cell carcinoma – unlike trichoepithelioma, demonstrates clefting, myxoid stroma, high nuclear:cytoplasmic ratio
>
> Microcystic adnexal carcinoma –may have ductular differentiation, perineural invasion, extension deep into reticular dermis or even subcutis
>
> Syringoma – no follicular differentiation, well-circumscribed, dense, and sclerotic stroma surrounds small ductules

- Trichoadenoma (Figs. 5.6 and 5.7)

  - Best regarded as "well-differentiated" trichoepithelioma

    o Rare, usually in adults
    o Numerous horn cysts, lining of cysts with squamous cells with a single layer of granular cells (*resemble cysts in seborrheic keratoses*)
    o Foreign body giant cells common

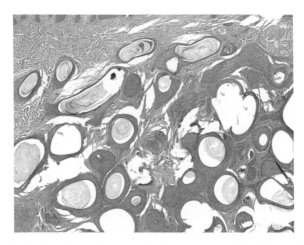

Fig. 5.6 Trichoadenoma is a dermal neoplasm composed of islands of keratinocytes showing pronounced follicular differentiation with well-formed cysts lined by granular keratinocytes. Original magnification ×40

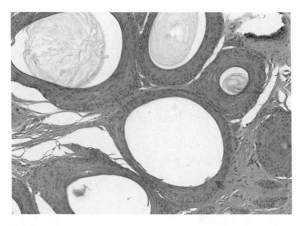

Fig. 5.7 Horned cysts lined by keratinocytes with prominent keratohyalin granules are present in trichoadenomas. Original magnification ×200

- Trichoblastoma

  - Clinical

    o Best regarded as "poorly differentiated" form of trichoepithelioma
    o Single nodule, often on scalp in adults
    o Some believe basaloid tumors arising from nevus sebaceus of Jadassohn, previously thought to be basal cell carcinomas, are all trichoblastomas

  - Histologic (Figs. 5.8, 5.9, and 5.10)

    o Well-circumscribed proliferation of basaloid, immature cells
    o Poor peripheral palisading
    o Minimal cleft formation
    o Papillary mesenchymal bodies and other follicular differentiation – less florid than in trichoepithelioma, but present more frequently than in basal cell carcinoma

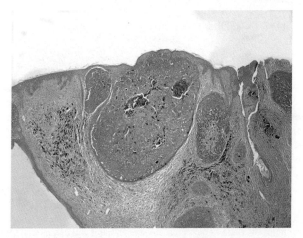

Fig. 5.8 Trichoblastoma is comprised of basaloid cells with only focal follicular differentiation. The surrounding stroma is adherent to the basaloid islands without clefting artifact seen in basal cell carcinomas. Original magnification ×40

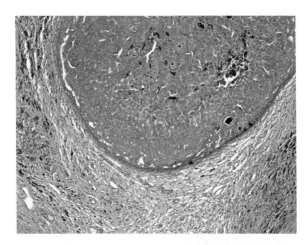

Fig. 5.9 There is little stromal separation from the epithelial islands in trichoblastoma, helping to differentiate these neoplasms from basal cell carcinoma. Pigment is often present. Original magnification ×100

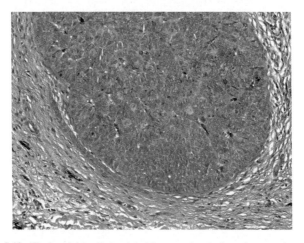

Fig. 5.10 The basaloid cells in trichoblastoma do not show the same degree of palisading or overlapping nuclei as are seen in basal cell carcinoma. Original magnification ×200

o Variable degrees of accompanying stroma – more fibrotic and less myxoid than basal cell carcinoma stroma (trichoblastic fibroma is variant of trichoblastoma with abundant stromal component)

o "rippled" variant with characteristic histologic appearance of alternating ribbons of epithelial nests and stroma (Fig. 5.11)

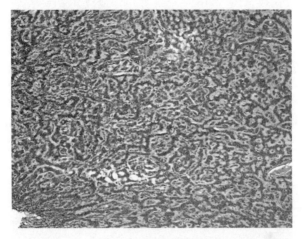

Fig. 5.11 A rippled trichoblastoma shows cells similar to those seen in pigmented trichoblastomas, but with cords of epithelial cells coursing between parallel bundles of collagen, giving rise to a rippled appearance. Original magnification ×100

• Pilomatricoma

– Clinical

o Firm, deep-seated nodule covered by skin
o Can be red-blue in color
o Usually solitary on face and upper extremities
o 40% in children <10 years old
o Multiple associated with myotonic dystrophy (very rare)

– Histologic (Figs. 5.12, 5.13, 5.14, 5.15, and 5.16)

o Centered in lower dermis
o Basophilic cells and shadow cells

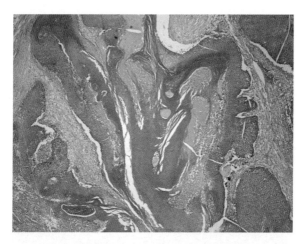

Fig. 5.12 Pilomatricomas are comprised of areas with marked proliferations of basaloid cells adjacent to very eosinophilic areas comprised of "shadow" cells. Original magnification ×40

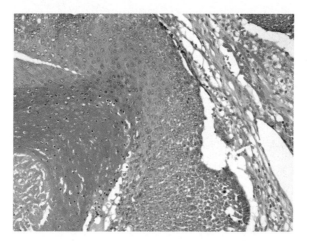

Fig. 5.13 Pilomatricomas demonstrate areas of abrupt keratinization with the basaloid cells merging immediately into the areas with "shadow" cells, with no granular layer present. Original magnification ×200

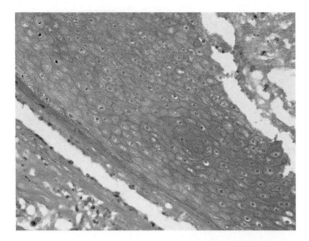

Fig. 5.14 "Shadow" or "ghost" cells, keratinocytes lacking their nuclei, are characteristic in pilomatricomas. Original magnification ×400

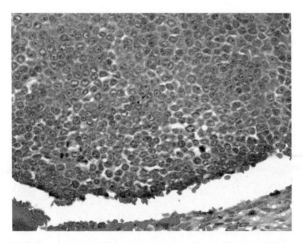

Fig. 5.15 Pilomatricomas demonstrate sheets of basaloid cells with prominent nucleoli within vesicular nuclei. Abundant mitoses may be present in these regions. Original magnification ×400

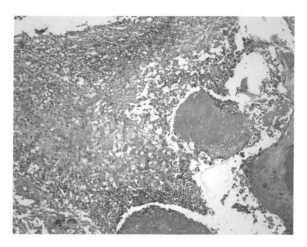

Fig. 5.16 Granulation tissue and marked inflammation may be present in ruptured areas of pilomatricoma. Original magnification ×400

- o   Older lesions with fewer basaloid cells
- o   Shadow cells – keratinocytes that have lost nuclei
- o   Abundant mitoses (none atypical)
- o   Abrupt keratinization (no granular layer)
- o   Calcification and giant cell reaction quite common
- o   Malignant variant – rare – adults, large size, marked atypia, excessive atypical mitoses, infiltrative growth pattern, zonal necrosis

- Trichilemmoma

  - Clinical

    - o   Usually single – quite common
    - o   Skin-colored, dome-shaped papule
    - o   May have tuft of hair emanating from central dell
    - o   Multiple associated with Cowden's syndrome (multiple hamartoma syndrome)

      Autosomal dominant
      Breast carcinoma

Fibrous hamartomas of breast, thyroid, GI tract
pTEN mutation

- Histologic (Figs. 5.17 and 5.18)

  o Acanthotic proliferation extending down from overlying epidermis
  o Centered around hair follicle
  o Tumor cells with abundant glycogen-rich clear cytoplasm
  o Thickened basement membrane zone recapitulating outer root sheath differentiation
  o Basal keratinocytes with clearing and peripheral palisade (but no clefting and no increase in nuclear:cytoplasmic ratio)
  o Hypergranulosis
  o Often parakeratosis over central portion of lesion– Desmoplastic variant described with central portion of lesion demonstrating abundant stroma interspersed with

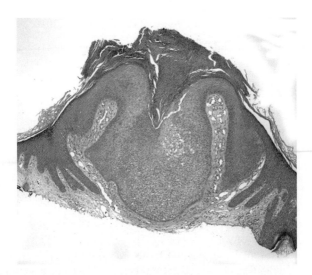

Fig. 5.17 Trichilemmoma appears as a cup-shaped, symmetrical lesion growing down from the epidermis. The cells demonstrate a characteristic pallor to the cytoplasm. Original magnification ×40

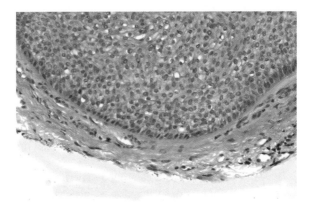

Fig. 5.18 There is palisading of the basal layer of cells rimming trichilemmoma, and often the basement membrane appears thickened under these areas. Original magnification ×200

smaller nests of keratinocytes with trichilemmal differentiation – *can be difficult to distinguish from basal cell or squamous cell carcinoma* (Figs. 5.19 and 5.20)

- Proliferating trichilemmal tumor
  - Clinical
    - o Usually single nodule without epidermal changes
    - o 90% on scalp
    - o >80% occurs in women
    - o May ulcerate and resemble SCC
    - o May arise from trichilemmal (pilar; isthmus/catagen) cysts
  - Histologic (Figs. 5.21, 5.22, and 5.23)
    - o Lobules of squamous epithelium, some with pale, glassy cytoplasm
    - o Abrupt keratinization as in trichilemmal cysts (i.e., no granular layer separating keratin from nucleated keratinocytes in areas of keratinization)
    - o Some horn cysts, squamous eddies
    - o Differs from squamous cell carcinoma by

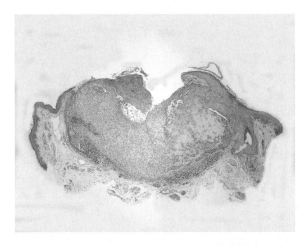

Fig. 5.19 Desmoplastic trichilemmoma demonstrates the same low-power architectural features as seen in trichilemmoma but with central foci of desmoplasia. Original magnification ×40

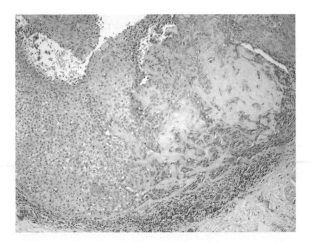

Fig. 5.20 Areas of desmoplastic stroma separate islands of pale staining keratinocytes in desmoplastic trichilemmomas. These areas are within the midst of the lesion and not at the deep margins. Original magnification ×100

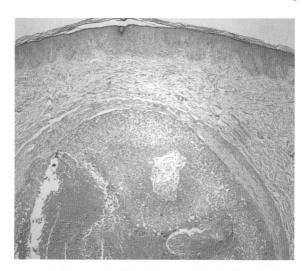

Fig. 5.21 Proliferating trichilemmal tumors are well-circumscribed dermal proliferations that have sharp, expanding margins. Original magnification ×40

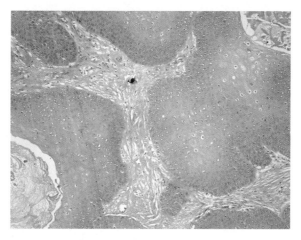

Fig. 5.22 Islands of bland appearing keratinocytes demonstrating abrupt keratinization (no granular layer prior to keratin formation) are present as papillomatous infoldings within the cystic structure in proliferating trichilemmal tumors. Original magnification ×100

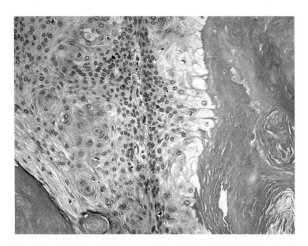

Fig. 5.23 Abrupt keratinization is characteristic of proliferating trichilemmal tumors. Mild cytologic atypia is sometimes present. Original magnification ×200

Only slight nuclear anaplasia
Sharp demarcation from surrounding stroma
Abrupt keratinization
Well-circumscribed

- o Rare malignant transformation
- o Some recent authors propose that all of these tumors are low-grade malignant neoplasms – *controversial*!

- Fibrofolliculoma

  - Clinical

    - o Non-descript papule/nodule, often on face
    - o Birt-Hogg-Dube syndrome – multiple fibrofolliculomas, trichodiscomas, and acrochordons – also associated with renal oncocytomas

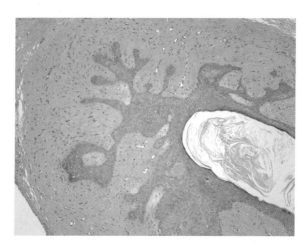

Fig. 5.24 Fibrofolliculoma is characterized by a central hair follicle that demonstrates thin islands of basaloid cells emanating from the central structure and surrounding dense fibrotic stroma. Original magnification ×100

- Histologic (Fig. 5.24)

   o Dermal tumor with well-circumscribed, dense stroma comprised of collagen bundles and small amounts of admixed mucin
   o Stromal is relatively hypercellular
   o Long cords of keratinocytes 3–4 cells in thickness with follicular differentiation interanastamose and course between the dense collagen bundles
   o *Some histologic resemblance to fibroadenoma of the breast*

- Trichodiscoma

   - Clinical

      o asymptomatic papules – may be single or multiple
      o often on face
      o may be identical to fibrofolliculomas (as per some authors)
      o associated with Birt-Hogg-Dube syndrome

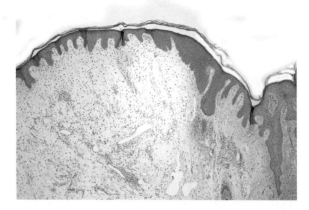

Fig. 5.25 Trichodiscoma is characterized by a well-circumscribed, non-encapsulated proliferation of mesenchymal cells embedded in myxoid stroma surrounded laterally by small hair follicles. Original magnification ×40

- Histologic (Fig. 5.25)
    - circumscribed, but not encapsulated growth of mesenchymal tissue that surrounds hair follicles
    - fascicles of fibrillar stroma admixed with myxoid ground substance
    - increased vascularity within stromal component
    - surrounded on either side of growth by distorted hair follicles (forming lateral borders of stromal growth)

- Tumor of the follicular infundibulum

    - Clinical
        - single plaque or nodule most common on head or neck
        - rarely associated with Cowden's syndrome
        - may occur in nevus sebaceus of Jadassohn

    - Histologic (Figs. 5.26 and 5.27)
        - grows down from overlying epidermis as plate-like inter-anastamosing of basaloid cells
        - slight palisading of peripheral cells in some cases

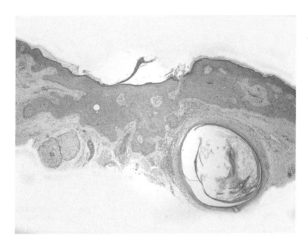

Fig. 5.26 Tumor of the follicular infundibulum grows as a plate-like proliferation comprised of interanastamosing cords of basaloid cells growing parallel to the epidermis. Original magnification ×40

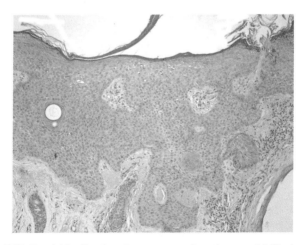

Fig. 5.27 Basaloid cells often demonstrate various degrees of follicular differentiation in tumors of the follicular infundibulum. Original magnification ×100

- o   aborted hair follicles and sebaceous glands may be seen
- o   these tumors have been described as having focal apocrine and sebaceous differentiation

- Tumors with sebaceous differentiation

  – Nevus sebaceus of Jadassohn
  – Sebaceous hyperplasia
  – Sebaceous adenoma
  – Sebaceoma (sebaceous epithelioma)
  – Sebaceous carcinoma

- Muir–Torre Syndrome (MTS)

  – Association of multiple sebaceous tumors and multiple visceral malignancies

    o   Does not include sebaceous hyperplasia or nevus sebaceus of Jadassohn as per most authors

  – Keratoacanthomas also part of MTS
  – Colon cancer and polyps – most common visceral involvement
  – Most visceral and cutaneous malignancies associated with MTS are low grade

- Nevus sebaceus of Jadassohn (NSJ)

  – Clinical

    o   Lesion on scalp or face, usually present at birth
    o   During childhood, only slightly raised, hairless plaque
    o   Enlarges during puberty and becomes nodular and yellow – much more prominent
    o   Can be associated with neurocutaneous syndrome – central nervous system – anomalies (very rare)

  – Histologic (Figs. 5.28, 5.29, 5.30, 5.31, and 5.32)

    o   Difficult to diagnose pre-pubertal as sebaceous glands not well-developed (can be diagnosed based upon clinical presentation, epidermal hyperplasia without atypia, lack of terminal hairs, apocrinization of eccrine glands)

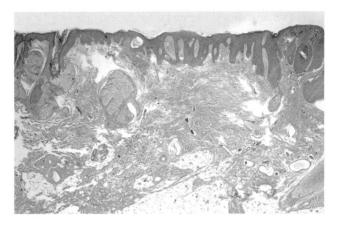

Fig. 5.28 Nevus sebaceus of Jadassohn (NSJ) demonstrates areas devoid of a mature hair growth. Original magnification ×20

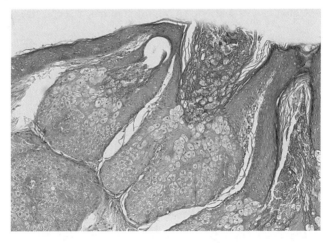

Fig. 5.29 In NSJ, sebaceous glands demonstrate abnormal insertion directly into the overlying epidermis. Original magnification ×100

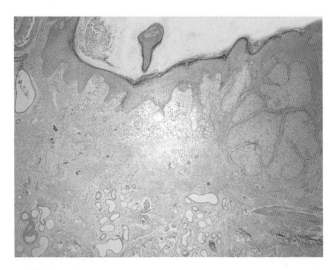

Fig. 5.30 Apocrinization of dermal glandular structures is characteristic of NSJ. Original magnification ×40

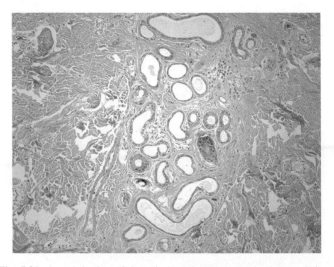

Fig. 5.31 Apocrinization of dermal glandular structures is characteristic of NSJ. Original magnification ×100

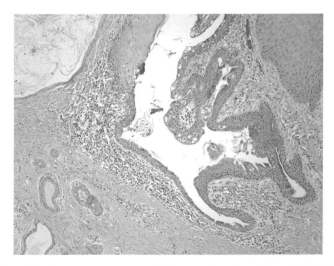

Fig. 5.32 Syringocystadenoma papilliferum often arises from within NSJ. Original magnification ×100

- o At puberty, many large, well-formed sebaceous glands opening directly to surface
- o Epidermal hyperplasia and papillomatosis
- o Hairs small, poorly formed
- o Ectopic apocrine glands (or apocrine metaplasia) in about 65% of cases

• Associated tumors

  – Syringocystadenoma papilliferum – found in 8–19% of cases
  – Less commonly

  - o Nodular hidradenoma
  - o Syringoma
  - o Sebaceous epithelioma
  - o Chondroid syringoma
  - o Trichilemmoma

- Trichoblastoma (previously thought to be BCC) present in 5–7% of cases
- SCC, apocrine carcinoma, porocarcinoma rare

- Sebaceous hyperplasia
  - Clinical
    - Forehead and cheeks of elderly patients
    - Elevated 2–3 mm yellow papules
  - Histologic (Figs. 5.33 and 5.34)
    - Single enlarged gland with multiple lobules grouped around central duct
    - Mature appearing, with only scant basaloid cells along periphery
    - Proliferation rate of sebocytes is slower than normal, not increased

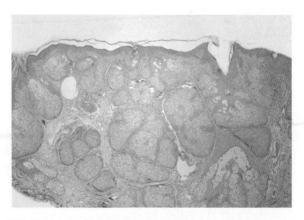

Fig. 5.33 Sebaceous hyperplasia demonstrates an increased number of enlarged sebaceous glands demonstrating complete maturation. Original magnification ×40

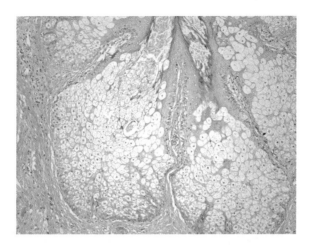

Fig. 5.34 Complete maturation with only a single layer of basaloid keratinocytes is seen in sebaceous hyperplasia. Original magnification ×100

- Sebaceous adenoma
  - Clinical
    - o Yellow papule/nodule
  - Histologic (Figs. 5.35 and 5.36)
    - o Sharply demarcated proliferation of incompletely differentiated sebocytes
    - o Undifferentiated basaloid cells at periphery of lobules surround centrally located sebocytes
    - o Basaloid cells comprise up to 50% of total cells in tumor
    - o See foci of keratinization
    - o Ones with cystic cavities in center more intimately associated with MTS (Fig. 5.37)

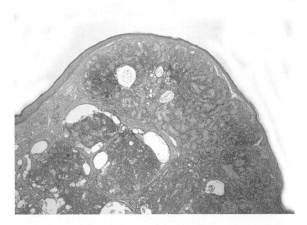

Fig. 5.35 Sebaceous adenomas demonstrate lobules of keratinocytes with sebaceous differentiation and admixed basaloid cells comprising less than 50% of the islands. Original magnification ×40

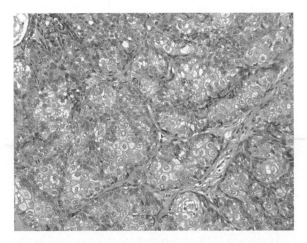

Fig. 5.36 Basaloid cells and mature sebocytes are admixed within lobules in sebaceous adenoma. Original magnification ×200

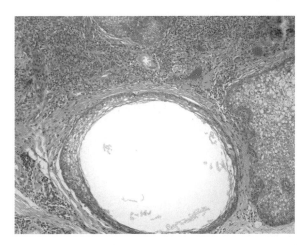

Fig. 5.37 Sebaceous adenomas containing cystic spaces in the sebaceous lobules are commonly associated with Muir–Torre syndrome. Original magnification ×100

- Sebaceoma

  - Histologic (Figs. 5.38 and 5.39)

    o Essentially synonymous with sebaceous epithelioma
    o Basal cells around periphery of lobules comprise more than 50% of tumor cells
    o Sebocytic differentiation prominent in center of lobules
    o Do not metastasize

- Sebaceous carcinoma

  - Clinical

    o Most common on eyelids in meibomian glands
    o Less common in Zeis glands
    o Eyelid lesions metastasize – up to 22% in one study
    o Lesions in MTS are much more indolent than sporadically occurring sebaceous carcinomas
    o Eyelid sebaceous carcinomas associated with higher rate of metastasis than similar tumors occurring on other body sites

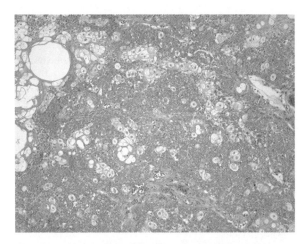

Fig. 5.38 Sebaceomas consist of lobules of basaloid cells with focal sebocytic differentiation. The basaloid cells are the major component and resemble those cells seen in basal cell carcinoma. Original magnification ×100

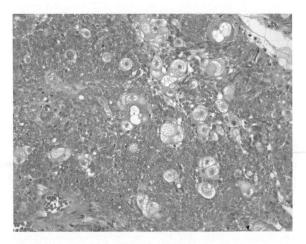

Fig. 5.39 Sebaceomas demonstrate minimal cytologic atypia but some degree of mitotic activity within the basaloid component. Original magnification ×200

- Histologic (Table 5.1, Figs. 5.40, 5.41, 5.42, and 5.43)

  o Great variation in size of tumor lobules
  o Many undifferentiated cells, usually only scattered cells
     with full sebocytic differentiation
  o Marked nuclear anaplasia, mitoses abundant
  o Pagetoid extension common

Table 5.1 Differential diagnosis of Pagetoid cells

–   Melanoma
–   Nevus – traumatized, congenital, recurrent, nevus of special sites
–   Squamous cell carcinoma
–   Sebaceous carcinoma
–   Porocarcinoma
–   Paget's disease
–   Extramammary Paget's disease

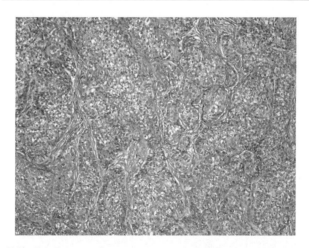

Fig. 5.40 Sebaceous carcinomas are composed of basaloid cells with focal
sebocytic differentiation and are atypical and pleomorphic. Lobular architecture may not be present. Original magnification ×100

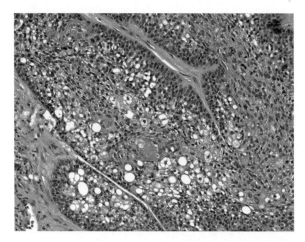

Fig. 5.41 In well-differentiated sebaceous carcinomas, sebocytic differentiation may be quite apparent. Original magnification ×200

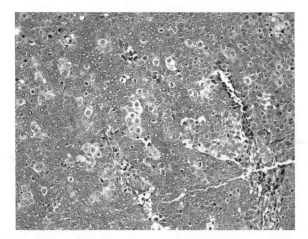

Fig. 5.42 In sebaceous carcinomas with poor differentiation, sebocytic differentiation is more focal, and immature, atypical keratinocytes make up the majority of the lesion. Original magnification ×200

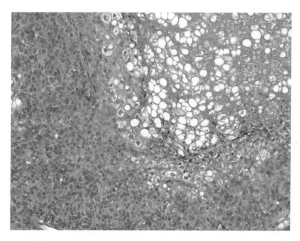

Fig. 5.43 Sebaceous carcinomas often demonstrate areas with zonal necrosis, a feature not seen in benign sebaceous neoplasms. Original magnification ×200

Chapter 6
Tumors with Eccrine Differentiation

- Large cell eccrine tumors (Table 6.1)

    - Eccrine acrospiroma

        o Poroma – arises from epidermis and extends into dermis
        o Dermal duct tumor – no connection to epidermis, tumor in papillary dermis and superficial reticular dermis
        o Hidradenoma – predominantly reticular dermal tumor

- Eccrine poroma

    - Clinical

        o common tumor – 2/3 on soles or sides of feet
        o usually arises in middle-aged people
        o firm, slightly pedunculated tumor
        o often with clinical appearance of vascular neoplasm (highly vascular component is clinically apparent)

    - Histology (Figs. 6.1 and 6.2)

        o tumor mass extends down from lower portion of epidermis in broad, anastamosing bands
        o cells have cuboidal appearance with small dark nuclei and abundant cytoplasmic glycogen
        o no keratin within tumor, can be hyperkeratotic or parakeratotic at surface

B.R. Smoller, K.M. Hiatt, *Epidermal Cell Tumors: The Basics*,
DOI 10.1007/978-1-4419-7704-5_6,
© Springer Science+Business Media, LLC 2011

Table 6.1 Tumors with eccrine differentiation

Large cell tumors (acrospiromas)
Eccrine poroma/porocarcinoma
Hidradenoma/hidradenocarcinoma
Dermal duct tumor
Small cell tumors
Spiradenoma/spiradenocarcinoma
Cyindroma/cylindromatous carcinoma
Tumors with ductular differentiation
Syringoma
Chondroid syringoma/malignant chondroid carcinoma
Microcystic carcinoma
Syringomatous carcinoma

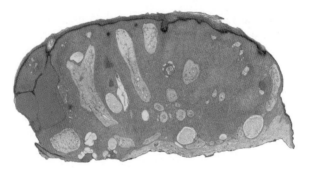

Fig. 6.1 Eccrine poroma shows a proliferation of keratinocytes extending in broad bands from the overlying epidermis

- o no palisading at periphery of tumoral islands (unlike basal cell carcinoma, some follicular neoplasms)
- o widely ectatic vessels in papillary dermis
- o ductular lumina lined by PAS+ cuticles
- o may see reduplicated basement membrane (hyalinized material) within tumor mass
- o *hidroacanthoma simplex* – eccrine poroma confined to entirely within epidermis

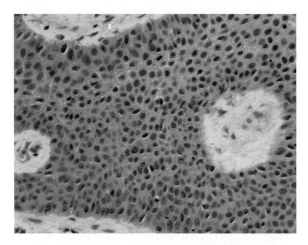

Fig. 6.2 High power of an eccrine poroma shows regular nuclei with abundant cytoplasm. Peripheral palisading is not present in a poroma

- Eccrine porocarcinoma (Figs. 6.3, 6.4, and 6.5)

  - Rare, usually arises from long-standing eccrine poromas, but can arise de novo
  - Can metastasize and result in death
  - Pagetoid cells seen in porocarcinomas (but not common in poromas)
  - Infiltrative growth pattern within dermis
  - Atypical mitoses
  - Necrotic cells abundant – areas of zonal necrosis

- Hidradenoma

  - Clinical

    o relatively common tumor
    o no site predilection
    o intradermal nodules with no overlying surface changes
    o usually single

  - Histology (Figs. 6.6, 6.7, 6.8, 6.9, and 6.10)

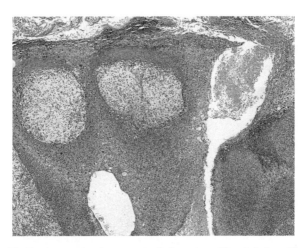

Fig. 6.3 Eccrine porocarcinoma extends from the epidermis in broad bands, similar to its benign counterpart

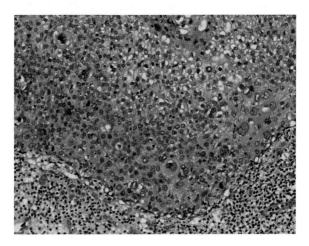

Fig. 6.4 Atypia and mitoses are prevalent in eccrine porocarcinoma

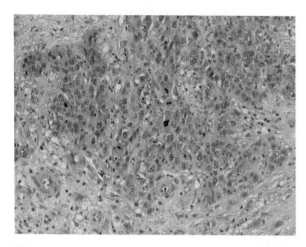

Fig. 6.5 Eccrine porocarcinoma has an infiltrative border as well as cytologic atypia and atypical mitoses

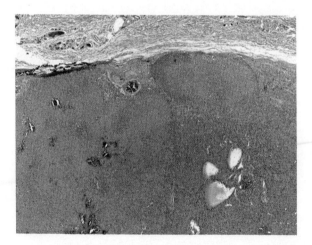

Fig. 6.6 Hidradenoma is a well-circumscribed dermal nodule which when solid may have a vague nodularity

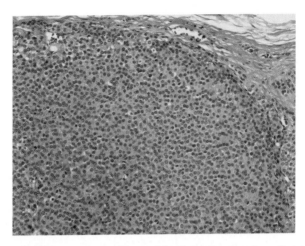

Fig. 6.7 Hidradenoma has uniform nuclei and abundant cytoplasm. Peripheral palisading is not present and occasional ductules may be noted

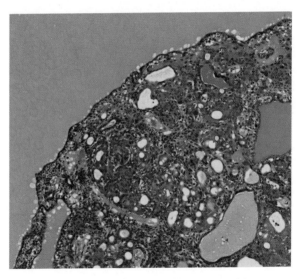

Fig. 6.8 This cystic variant of hidradenoma shows a nest with numerous small cystic spaces within a much larger cystic space

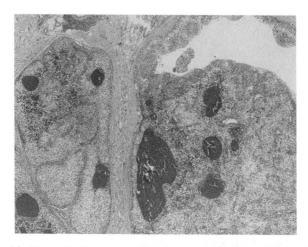

Fig. 6.9 Clear cell hidradenoma shows the same well-circumscribed lobular architecture as the conventional variant and may also have cystic spaces as in this lesion

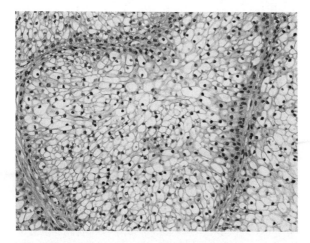

Fig. 6.10 Higher power of this clear cell hidradenoma shows abundant glycogenated cytoplasm and uniform, small nuclei

- o well-circumscribed dermal nodule – usually in reticular dermis
- o lobules of keratinocytes with rare luminal differentiation
- o cystic spaces may be present and may contain eccrine secretions
- o may extend into subcutaneous fat
- o uniform appearance to tumor cells: some small and dark, others a bit larger with more open appearing nuclei
- o clear cell change common – due to increased cytoplasmic glycogen
- o focal squamous differentiation seen occasionally
- o reduplicated basement membrane (hyalinized) a common feature
- o does not connect to epidermis (in ideal world – small foci of connection not uncommon)

- Hidradenocarcinoma (Fig. 6.11)

  - Rare neoplasms
  - Usually arise de novo as malignant tumors
  - High rate of metastasis and death

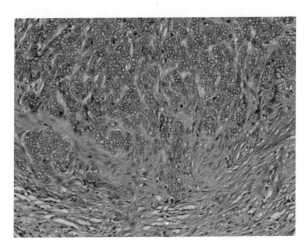

Fig. 6.11 Hidradenocarcinoma is characterized by an infiltrate margin in a nodule composed of cells with large nuclei and frequent mitoses

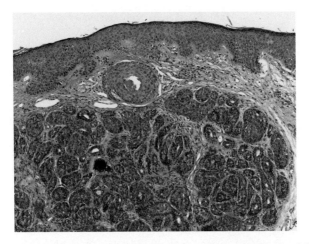

Fig. 6.12 Dermal duct tumor is composed of a well-circumscribed nodule in the superficial dermis. Duct formation is typically prevalent

- Infiltrative growth pattern
- High mitotic rate with atypical figures
- Zonal necrosis
- Vascular invasion

- Dermal duct tumor (Fig. 6.12)

  - Identical to hidradenoma but located primarily in papillary and superficial reticular dermis

- Small cell eccrine tumors

  - Eccrine spiradenoma
  - Cylindroma

- Eccrine spiradenoma

  - Clinical

    o arise in early adulthood
    o usually 1–2 cm solitary intradermal nodule
    o characteristically painful (Table 6.2)

  - Histology (Figs. 6.13 and 6.14)

Table 6.2 Painful dermal tumors

Blue rubber bleb nevus

Leiomyoma
Eccrine spiradenoma
Neurilemmoma (dermal schwannoma)
Dercum's disease (adiposa dolorosa)
Angiolipoma/angiomyolipoma
Neuroma, neurofibroma
Endometriosis
Glomus tumor
Granular cell tumor
Osteoma cutis/calcinosis cutis

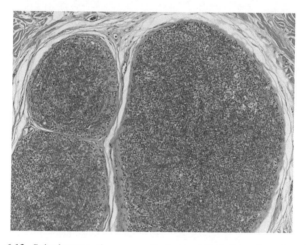

Fig. 6.13 Spiradenoma shows a well-circumscribed deep dermal nodule composed of two cell types

- ○ well-circumscribed dermal nodules without connection to epidermis
- ○ two cell types: cells with small dark nuclei
  cells with slightly larger, more vesicular nuclei (more numerous)
- ○ PAS+ lumina usually present (also CEA+, cytokeratin 7+)
- ○ reduplicated basement membrane (type IV collagen) present between epithelial cells

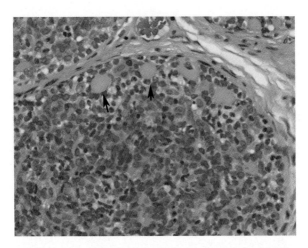

Fig. 6.14 High power of spiradenoma shows a population of larger cells with larger, vesicular nuclei and a small population of smaller cells with small hyperchromatic nuclei. Reduplicated basement membrane (*arrows*) is commonly found in eccrine tumors

- o malignant degeneration of long-standing lesions has been reported to result in death in rare patients
- o spiradenocarcinomas have marked anaplasia, mitoses, and necrosis

- Cylindroma
  - Clinical
    - o usually single
    - o autosomal dominantly inherited tends to be multiple and is often referred to as "turban tumors"
    - o appears in adulthood
    - o frequent association of multiple cylindromas and multiple trichoepitheliomas (Brooke–Spiegler syndrome)
    - o also rarely associated with eccrine spiradenoma

  - Histology (Figs. 6.15 and 6.16)
    - o numerous islands of epithelial cells surrounded by hyaline sheaths and collagen

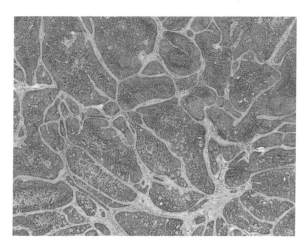

Fig. 6.15 Cylindromas are composed of well-circumscribed dermal nodules made up of numerous islands of epithelial cells that fit together like the spots on a giraffe

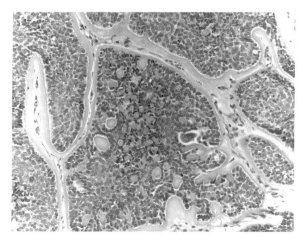

Fig. 6.16 This high-power image of a cylindroma demonstrates the two cell types, similar to that seen in spiradenoma, that make the islands. Also present is the eosinophilic amorphous material representing reduplicated basement membrane

- islands fit together like "pieces of a jigsaw puzzle"
- two cell types in islands of cells (cells with small dark nuclei and other cells with larger, more vesicular nuclei – identical to cell types seen in spiradenoma)
- occasional tubular lumina
- rare malignant transformation characterized by anaplasia, mitoses, and invasion of local tissue (malignant degeneration almost always in patients with multiple cylindromas)

- Tumors with acrosyringeal differentiation

  - Syringoma
  - Chondroid syringoma (and malignant)

- Eccrine carcinoma

  - Microcystic adnexal carcinoma

- Syringoma
  - Clinical

    - more common in women
    - onset at puberty or later
    - 1–2 mm skin-colored papules
    - lower eyelids most common, also on vulva, axilla, abdomen
    - sudden onset of many referred to as "eruptive syringomas"
    - may be "malformations" and not true neoplasms

  - Histologic (Figs. 6.17, 6.18, and 6.19)

    - small ducts lined by two layers of cells coursing in densely fibrous stroma
    - comma-like or tadpole-like structures are characteristic
    - dilated cystic structures may occasionally keratin
    - restricted to papillary dermis
    - clear cell variant is associated with diabetes mellitus

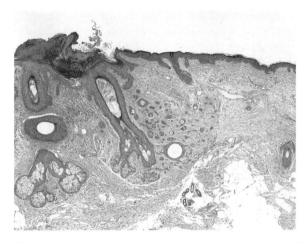

Fig. 6.17 This low-power image of a syringoma demonstrates that proliferation is restricted to the superficial dermis, without an infiltrate pattern to the deep aspect

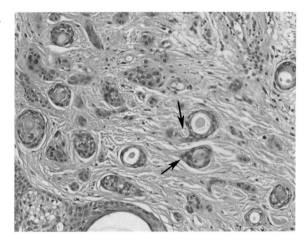

Fig. 6.18 Higher power of a syringoma demonstrates the two cell layers that make up the ductular structures. The characteristic "tadpole-like" morphology can be seen in some of the duct (*arrows*)

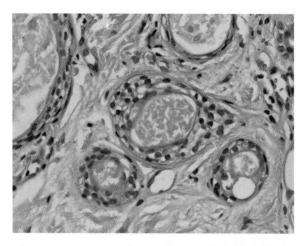

Fig. 6.19 This clear cell syringoma differs from the conventional type only by the more abundant clear cytoplasm of the cells making up the ductular structures

- ○ *differential diagnosis includes morpheaform basal cell carcinoma, microcystic adnexal carcinoma, and desmoplastic trichoepithelioma*

- Chondroid syringoma
  - Clinical
    - ○ indistinct dermal tumors
    - ○ most common on head and neck
    - ○ no clinical relationship with "syringoma"
    - ○ more common in males
    - ○ usually arise in middle age
    - ○ may be nosologically related to eccrine and/or apocrine structures
  - Histologic (Figs. 6.20, 6.21, and 6.22)
    - ○ tubules with branching or ductules embedded in mucinous stroma

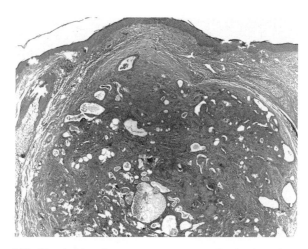

Fig. 6.20 Chondroid syringoma, or cutaneous mixed tumor, is a well-circumscribed dermal tumor composed of epithelial elements forming ducts and tubes lined by two cell layers, a myxoid stroma, and foci of chondroid differentiation, all well-represented in this lesion

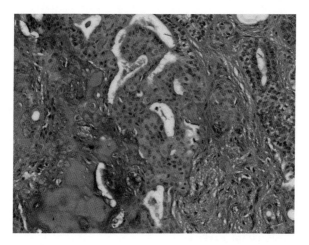

Fig. 6.21 Higher power of this chondroid syringoma shows approximately equal representation of the three components: epithelial, chondroid, and myxoid stroma

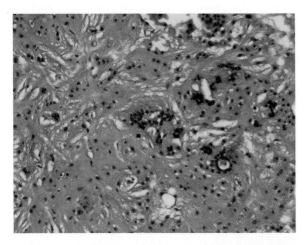

Fig. 6.22 This chondroid syringoma has only a small population of epithelial cells with abundant myxoid stroma and small foci of chondroid differentiation

- o ductules lined by cells identical to those seen in syringoma – two layers
  - o secretion may be present within ductular spaces
  - o stroma contains sulfated acid mucopolysaccharides (alcian blue and colloidal Fe positive at low pHs)
- Malignant chondroid syringoma (Fig. 6.23)
  - Very rare
  - Usually arises de novo as malignant neoplasms
  - Often on thighs
  - Can metastasize
  - Cells are atypical, poorly formed tubules
  - Mitoses, vascular invasion, necrosis seen
- Microcystic adnexal carcinoma
  - Clinical
    - o most on face between upper lip and lower eyelid
    - o appears as indurated, depressed scar-like lesion

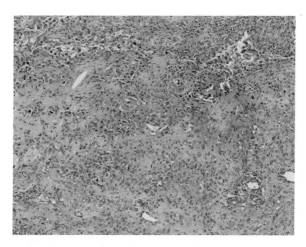

Fig. 6.23 Malignant mixed tumor loses definitive epithelial differentiation as demonstrated by the sheets of cells with significant cytologic atypia. Mitoses may also be seen

- o biopsies from these lesions usually submitted as "rule out scar vs. morpheic basal cell carcinoma" – *important that clinical presentation is very different from syringoma*

  - Histologic (Figs. 6.24, 6.25, and 6.26)

    - o biphasic differentiation (follicular and ductular) in many cases
    - o no cytologic atypia
    - o infiltrative growth pattern
    - o extend into deeper dermis and subcutaneous fat
    - o perineural invasion common
    - o rare (if any) reported cases of metastasis

Other types of eccrine carcinoma (Table 6.3)

- Less common tumors with eccrine differentiation

  - Eccrine nevus
  - Eccrine syringofibroadenoma
  - Mucinous syringometaplasia

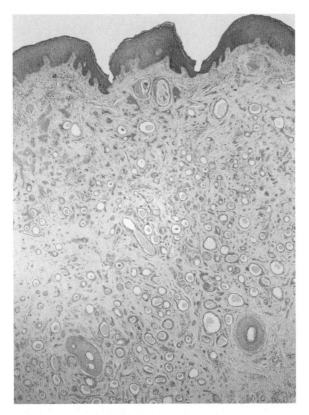

Fig. 6.24 Microcystic adnexal carcinoma is a deeply infiltrative tumor composed of benign appearing epithelial elements showing eccrine and follicular differentiation

- Papillary eccrine (or apocrine) adenoma
- Eccrine nevus (Figs. 6.27 and 6.28)
  - Defined as increased numbers of normal eccrine glands
  - May be associated with increased vascularity (and rarely also increased numbers of nerves) known as eccrine angiomatous hamartoma
- Syringofibroadenoma (Figs. 6.29 and 6.30)

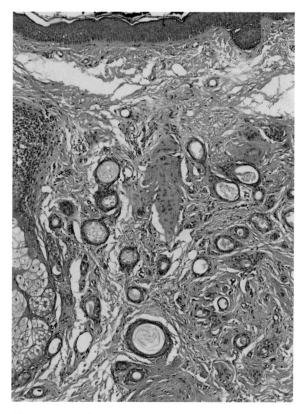

Fig. 6.25 This image of microcystic adnexal carcinoma shows ductules composed of two cell layers of cuboidal cells with deceptively bland small hyperchromatic nuclei

- Clinical

    o Solitary, hyperkeratotic papule or nodule on extremity
    o Similar changes can be seen adjacent to inflammatory conditions and are likely reactive changes

- Histologic

    o Interanastamosing cords of ductular epithelium with a plate-like growth pattern extending down from epidermis

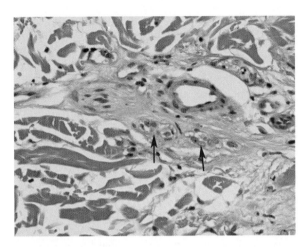

Fig. 6.26 This image shows small clusters of microcystic adnexal carcinoma (*arrows*) in the deep reticular dermis tracking along a small nerve

Table 6.3   Other types of eccrine carcinoma

Classic	Resembles other types of adenocarcinoma	High metastasis rate
Syringoid eccrine carcinoma	Resembles basal cell carcinoma with eccrine differentiation	Low metastasis rate
Mucinous eccrine carcinoma	Rare	Almost never metastasizes
Adenoid cystic carcinoma	Resembles salivary gland neoplasm; rarest subtype	Rarely metastasizes

- o Cells morphologically resemble those of eccrine poroma: small, central nuclei, often slightly clear cytoplasm
- o Vascular-rich stroma underlying epithelial proliferation
- Mucinous syringometaplasia
  - Reactive metaplastic condition
  - Crushed papules, usually on feet, hands
  - Mostly young men

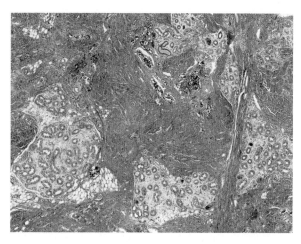

Fig. 6.27 Eccrine nevus is characterized by the numerous eccrine glands in the reticular dermis

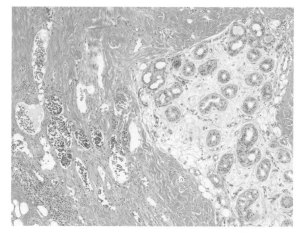

Fig. 6.28 In eccrine nevus, the eccrine glands have benign cytology. As in this case, there is often an associated vascular component. In this case, the lesion is more accurately referred to as an eccrine angiomatous nevus (hamartoma)

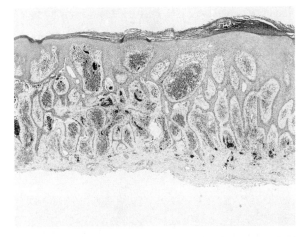

Fig. 6.29 Syringofibroadenoma shows extensive anastomosing of epithelial cords projecting from the epidermis. The cells have benign cytology and the stroma has numerous ectatic, thin-walled vessels

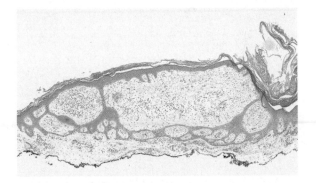

Fig. 6.30 In this syringofibroadenoma there is less abundant epithelial projections than in the lesion shown in Fig. 6.29. The lesion shows anastomosing of epithelial strands composed of benign cuboidal cells in a vascular-rich stroma

- – Squamous metaplasia of eccrine ducts from surface down to base

- Papillary eccrine adenoma

  - – Clinical

    - o Rare
    - o Usually on extremities
    - o Slightly more common in females
    - o May or may not be identical to tubular apocrine adenoma

  - – Histologic (Figs. 6.31 and 6.32)

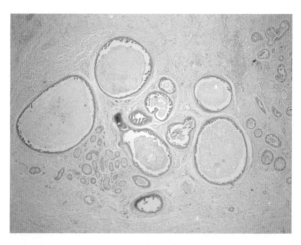

Fig. 6.31 This low-power image of a papillary eccrine adenoma shows the variability in the size of the ducts and cysts in this well-circumscribed dermal tumor

    - o Well-circumscribed tumor of branching ducts and cysts in dense stroma
    - o Papillary projections frequent

Tumors with apocrine differentiation (Table 6.4)

- Hidradenoma papilliferum

  - – Clinical

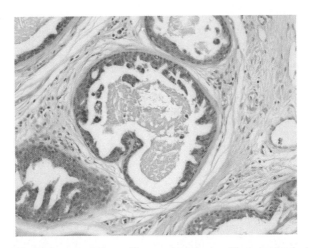

Fig. 6.32 Higher power of a papillary eccrine adenoma illustrates the duct lining composed of cuboidal epithelial cells with small nuclei. The lining forms papillary projections into the lumen. Eccrine secretions are often present in the lumen

Table 6.4   Tumors with apocrine differentiation

Hidradenoma papilliferum
Syringocystadenoma papilliferum
Cylindroma
Aprocrine adenoma
Tubular apocrine adenoma

- o Virtually always in women, on labia majora or in perineal or perianal region
- o Solitary nodule
- o Malignant transformation only reported in one patient (dubious – the associated malignancy was reported to be a squamous cell carcinoma)

– Histology (Figs. 6.33 and 6.34)

- o Well-circumscribed dermal tumor with no connection to overlying epidermis
- o Tubular and cystic structures with papillary infoldings

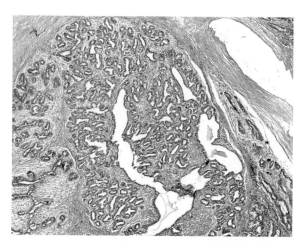

Fig. 6.33 This image of hidradenoma papilliferum shows a well-circumscribed lobule composed of numerous branching tubular structures

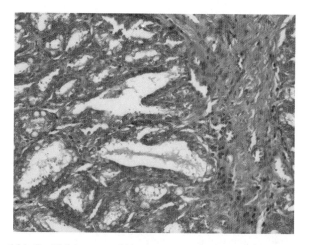

Fig. 6.34 On higher power, hidradenoma papilliferum shows the tubular structures lined by low cuboidal cells without pleomorphism or mitoses. Small papilla can be seen projecting into the lumen

- o Lumina surrounded by 1–2 layers of cells (epithelial and myoepithelial)
- o Fibrous collagen between epithelial proliferations
- o Not as inflammatory as syringocystadenoma papilliferum

- Syringocystadenoma papilliferum

    - Clinical

        - o Ulcerated, verrucous plaque, often chronic and non-healing
        - o Oozing and weeping often described
        - o 33% associated with nevus sebaceus of Jadassohn
        - o Often clinically mimics basal cell carcinoma
        - o Malignant transformation extremely rare (if at all)

    - Histology (Figs. 6.35 and 6.36)

        - o Epidermal papillomatosis with invaginations into dermis lined by squamous or glandular epithelium

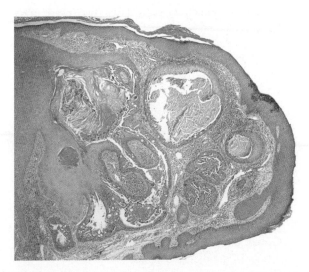

Fig. 6.35 Syringocystadenoma papilliferum is a dermal nodule composed of ducts that extend from the overlying epidermis. Squamatization of the ducts is noted near the surface

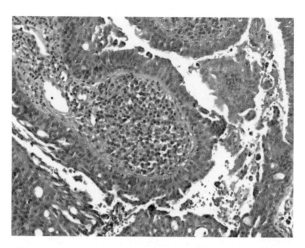

Fig. 6.36 The lining of the ducts in syringocystadenoma papilliferum varies from cuboidal to columnar. This papillary projection has thin-walled vessels and numerous plasma cells in its core

- Glandular epithelium consists of two rows of cells – luminal columnar cells and other cuboidal cells
- Connections with apocrine glands in the dermis can be found with step sections
- Dense infiltrate of plasma cells surrounding papillary infoldings
- 33% of total cases of these are associated with nevus sebaceus of Jadassohn
- Very rare malignant transformation with metastasis reported

- Aggressive digital papillary adenocarcinoma

  - Clinical

    - Ulcerated nodule located on fingers
    - Grows fairly rapidly
    - Tumor of middle-aged people
    - Histologic features do not correlate with clinical behavior; not advisable to label these lesions as adenoma based on benign cytology

- Treat all aggressively due to high rate of metastasis (up to 40%)/local recurrence (40%)
- Difficult to categorize as eccrine or apocrine neoplasm
- Metastasis most commonly to lung. Regional lymph nodes are second most common

- Histology (Figs. 6.37, 6.38, 6.39, and 6.40)

  - Surface most commonly ulcerated
  - Dense proliferation of glandular cells with papillary infoldings

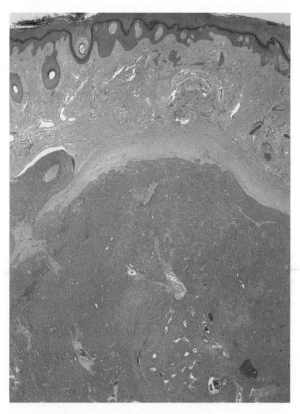

Fig. 6.37 Aggressive digital papillary adenocarcinoma is a dermal tumor without a connection to the overlying epidermis

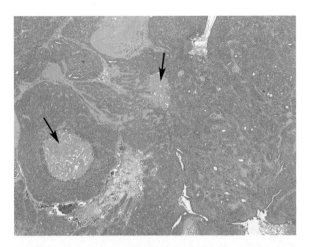

Fig. 6.38 The tumor in aggressive digital papillary adenocarcinoma grows as nests, glands, and nodules. Comedo-type necrosis (*arrows*) is common

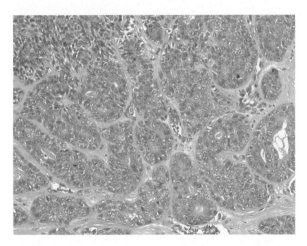

Fig. 6.39 While some areas of aggressive digital papillary adenocarcinoma cells form large sheets of tumor, other areas, such as this one, are formed by back-to-back glands with large nuclei, open chromatin, mitoses, and inspissated ductular secretions

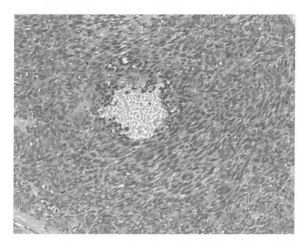

Fig. 6.40 Aggressive digital papillary adenocarcinoma may show numerous mitoses, nuclear pleomorphism, and necrosis, as in this image, or may have surprisingly benign cytology

- o Variable degrees of cytologic atypia, mitotic activity, necrosis (not predictive of clinical behavior)
- o Apocrine changes (eosinophilia, hobnail appearance) in some cases

Chapter 7
Merkel Cell Carcinoma

- Clinical features:

  - Sun-exposed head, neck, and upper extremities
  - Elderly patients (mean age 75), male predominance
  - Rarely in children
  - Red color often resembles angiosarcoma, but usually indistinguishable from other cutaneous neoplasms
  - Usually about 2 cm in diameter at time of presentation
  - Highly aggressive neoplasm
  - Incidence of 0.23/10,000 in Caucasian Americans, very rare in African Americans
  - 1500 new cases/year in USA – incidence rising rapidly

- Biological behavior:

  - Local recurrence in 25% of cases
  - Metastasis to regional nodes in 50% of cases
  - Distant metastases in 34% of cases
  - Death in 34% of cases

- Histologic features (Figs. 7.1, 7.2, 7.3, and 7.4):

  - Small round, uniform cells distributed in sheets and trabeculae
  - Vesicular nuclei, inconspicuous nucleoli
  - "Salt-and-pepper" chromatin
  - Minimal cytoplasm
  - Multiple mitoses and apoptotic cells

B.R. Smoller, K.M. Hiatt, *Epidermal Cell Tumors: The Basics*,   139
DOI 10.1007/978-1-4419-7704-5_7,
© Springer Science+Business Media, LLC 2011

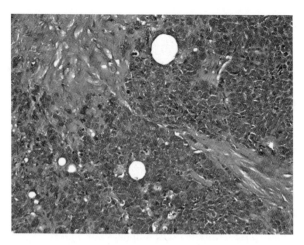

Fig. 7.1 Merkel cell carcinoma is characterized by sheets of dark cells coursing throughout the dermis. Original magnification ×100

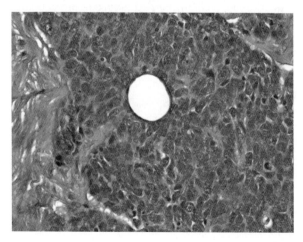

Fig. 7.2 The cells appear as dark nuclei with a salt-and-pepper chromatin pattern and only inconspicuous nucleoli. Original magnification ×200

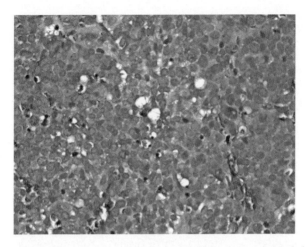

Fig. 7.3 Abundant apoptotic cells and mitotic activity are seen in Merkel cell carcinomas. Original magnification ×200

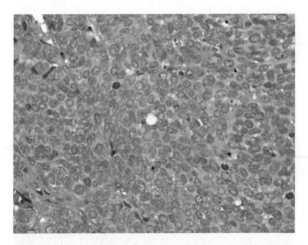

Fig. 7.4 The nuclei are often relatively pale staining, demonstrate dispersed chromatic patterns and minimal nucleoli in Merkel cell carcinoma. Original magnification ×200

- Epidermotropism in about 10% of cases (Figs. 7.5 and 7.6)
- Often areas with divergent differentiation (squamous cell carcinoma, basal cell carcinoma, rarely melanoma and fibrosarcoma) (Fig. 7.7)

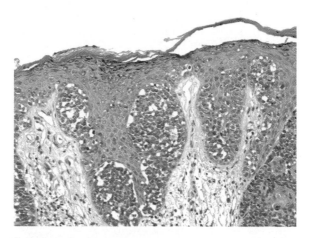

Fig. 7.5 Epidermotropism is seen in a significant minority of cases of Merkel cell carcinoma. Original magnification ×100

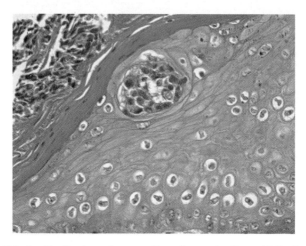

Fig. 7.6 Small collections of tumor cells can be seen in a Pagetoid distribution in some cases of Merkel cell carcinoma, raising the differential diagnosis of melanoma. Original magnification ×200

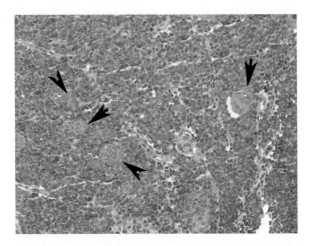

Fig. 7.7 Focal squamous differentiation (*arrows*) is frequently encountered in Merkel cell carcinoma. Original magnification ×100

- Immunohistochemical features:

  - Cytokeratin positive (dot-like pattern – paranuclear or membranous staining pattern) (Figs. 7.8 and 7.9)
  - Cytokeratin (CK)20 sensitive marker (not totally specific)
  - Thyroid transcription factor-1 (TTF-1) positive in small cell carcinomas of lung, but also rarely positive in Merkel cell carcinoma
  - Somatostatin and chromogranin frequently positive (Fig. 7.10)
  - Neuron-specific enolase (NSE) and epithelial membrane antigen (EMA) also positive but very non-specific
  - S100 negative

- Indicators of poor prognosis:

  - Male
  - Age >55 years
  - Location on head and neck
  - Advanced stage at time of diagnosis
  - Tumor >2 cm
  - Immunosuppression
  - Diffuse growth pattern

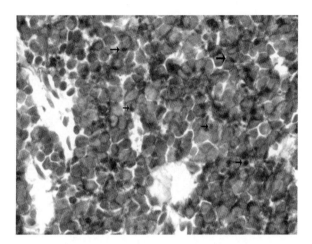

Fig. 7.8 Dot-like paranuclear staining (*arrows*) is characteristic of Merkel cell carcinoma stained with cytokeratin 20. Original magnification ×200

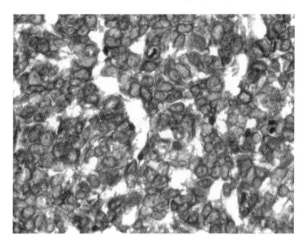

Fig. 7.9 A membranous pattern of staining with cytokeratin 20 can also be seen in Merkel cell carcinoma. Original magnification ×200

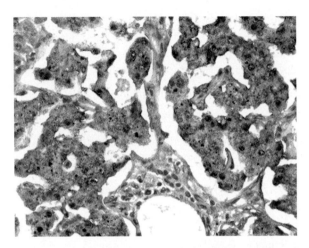

Fig. 7.10 Chromogranin stains Merkel cell carcinomas variably and often demonstrates high background staining. It is less reliable than the cytokeratin stains. Original magnification ×200

- Heavy lymphocytic infiltrate
- High mitotic rate
- P63 expression

- Merkel cell carcinoma – staging and prognosis:

  - 5-year survival rates:

    o Stage I: (T1 N0 M0 – primary tumor <2 cm) – 81%
    o Stage II: (T2 N0 M0 – primary tumor ≥2 cm) – 67%
    o Stage III: regional node involvement – 52%
    o Stage I: distant nodal involvement – 11%

- Etiology and pathogenesis

  - Probably *not* derived from cutaneous "Merkel" cells of the skin, but rather likely originates from pluripotent stem cells that undergo neuroendocrine differentiation
  - Strong association with presence of MC polyomavirus

- Virus found in integrated and clonal form in 70% of Merkel cell carcinoma
- Some cases are clearly negative, so not "necessary" for the development of Merkel cell carcinoma
- Cytogenetics and Merkel cell carcinoma:
  - Trisomy 6 present in >60% of cases of MCC, but not all
- Current treatments for Merkel cell carcinoma:
  - Wide local excision – standard therapy
    - <1 cm margins *not* associated with higher risk of recurrence
    - 2 cm margins best reserved for lesions >2 cm
  - Sentinel node (SN) biopsy – controversial
    - About 30% of patients have positive sentinel lymph nodes at time of presentation
  - Adjuvant post-operative radiation therapy – also controversial
  - Adjuvant chemotherapy of little use at this time – most Merkel cell carcinomas do not respond to standard chemotherapeutic regimens

Further Reading

Chapter 1

Common Acquired Melanocytic Nevus

Bauer J, Garbe C. Acquired melanocytic nevi as risk factor for melanoma development. A comprehensive review of epidemiologic data. Pigment Cell Res 2003; 16: 297–306.

Clemmensen OJ, Kroon S. The histology of "congenital features" in early acquired melanocytic nevi. J Am Acad Dermatol 1988; 19: 742–746.

Yus ES, del Cerro M, Simon RS, Herrera M, Rueda M. Unna's and Miescher's nevi: two different types of intradermal nevus: hypothesis concerning their histogenesis. Am J Dermatopathol 2007; 29: 141–151.

Congenital Nevus

Barnhill RL, Fleischli M. Histologic features of congenital melanocytic nevi in infants 1 year of age or younger. J Am Acad Dermatol 1995; 33: 780–785.

Tannous ZS, Mihm MC Jr, Sober AJ, Duncan LM. Congenital melanocytic nevi: clinical and histopathologic features, risk of melanoma, and clinical management. J Am Acad Dermatol 2005; 52: 197–203.

B.R. Smoller, K.M. Hiatt, *Epidermal Cell Tumors: The Basics*,
DOI 10.1007/978-1-4419-7704-5,
© Springer Science+Business Media, LLC 2011

Halo Nevus

Akasu R, From L, Kahn HJ. Characterization of the mononuclear infiltrate involved in regression of halo nevi. J Cutan Pathol 1994; 21: 302–311.

Zeff RA, Freitag A, Grin CM. Grant-Kels JM. The immune response in halo nevi. J Am Acad Dermatol 1997; 37: 620–624.

Nevus of Special Sites

Clark WH, Hood AF, Tucker MA, Jampel RM. Atypical melanocytic nevi of the genital type with a discussion of reciprocal parenchymal-stromal interactions in the biology of Neoplasia. Hum Pathol 1998; 29: S1–S24.

Hosler GA, Moresi JM, Barrett TL. Nevi with site-related atypia: a review of melanocytic nevi with atypical histologic features based upon anatomic site. J Cutan Pathol 2008; 35: 889–898.

Combined Nevus

Ball NJ, Golitz LE. Melanocytic nevi with focal atypical epithelioid cell components: a review of seventy-three cases. J Am Acad Dermatol 1994; 30: 724–729.

Scolyer RA, Zhuang L Palmer AA, Thompson JF, McCarthy SW. Combined naevus: a benign lesion frequently misdiagnosed both clinically and pathologically as melanoma. Pathology 2004; 36: 419–427.

Chapter 2

Malignant Melanoma

Byers HR, Bhawan J. Pathologic parameters in the diagnosis and prognosis of primary cutaneous melanoma. Hematol Oncol Clin North Am 1998; 12: 717–735.

Clark WH Jr, Evan HL, Everett MA, Farmer ER, Graham JH, Mihm MC Jr, Rosai J, Sagebiel RW, Wick MR. Early melanoma. Histologic terms. Am J Dermatopathol 1991; 13: 579–582.

Crowson AN, Magro CM, Mihm MC Jr. Prognosticators of melanoma, the melanoma report, and the sentinel lymph node. Mod Pathol 2006; 19 suppl 2: S71–S87.

Duncan LM. The classification of cutaneous melanoma. Hematol Oncol Clin North Am 2009; 23: 501–513.

Elder DE. Pathology of melanoma. Clin Cancer Res 2006; 12: 2308s–2311s.

Frishberg DP, Balch C, Balzer BL, Crowson AN, Didolkar M, McNiff JM, Perry RR, Prieto VG, Rao P, Smith MT, Smoller BR, Wick MR, Members of the Cancer Committee, College of American Pathologists. Protocol for the examination of specimens from patients with melanoma of the skin. Arch Pathol Lab Med 2009; 133: 1560–1567.

King R, Googe PB, Mihm MC Jr. Thin melanomas. Clin Lab Med 2000; 20: 713–729.

Mihm MC Jr, Clark WH Jr, From L. The clinical diagnosis, classification and histogenetic concepts of the early stages of cutaneous malignant melanoma. N Engl J Med 1971; 284: 1078–1082.

Pris A, Mihm MC Jr. Progress in melanoma histopathology and diagnosis. Hematol Oncol Clin North Am 2009; 23: 467–480.

Taran JM. Heenan PJ. Clinical and histologic features of level 2 cutaneous malignant melanoma associated with metastasis. Cancer 2001; 91: 1822–1825.

Chapter 3

Dysplastic (Atypical, Clark's) Nevus

Ackerman AB. Mythology and numerology in the sphere of melanoma. Cancer 2000; 88: 491–496.

Ackerman AB, Elder DE. An exchange of ideas about dysplastic nevi and malignant melanomas. Am J Dermatopathol 1985; 7 suppl: 99–105.

Black WC, Hunt WC. Histologic correlations with the clinical diagnosis of dysplastic nevus. Am J Surg Pathol 1990; 14(1): 44–52.

Cooke KR, Spear GF, Elder DE, Greene MH. Dysplastic naevi in a population-based survey. Cancer 1989; 63(6): 1240–1244.

Duncan LM, Berwick M, Bruijn JA, Byers HR, Mihm MC, Barnhill RL. Histopathologic recognition and grading of dysplastic melanocytic nevi: an interobserver agreement study. J Invest Dermatol 1993; 100: 318S–321S.

Hussein MR. Melanocytic dysplastic naevi occupy the middle ground between benign melanocytic naevi and cutaneous malignant melanomas: emerging clues. J Clin Pathol 2005; 58: 453–456.

Kelly JW, Crutcher WA, Sagebiel RW. Clinical diagnosis of dysplastic melanocytic nevi. A clinicopathologic correlation. J Am Acad Dermatol 1986; 14(6): 1044–1052.

Rabkin MS. The limited specificity of histological examination in the diagnosis of dysplastic nevi. J Cutan Pathol 2008; 35 suppl 2: 20–23.

Rhodes AR, Mihm MC Jr, Weinstock MA. Dysplastic melanocytic nevi: a reproducible histologic definition emphasizing cellular morphology. Mod Pathol 1989; 2(4): 306–319.

Spindle and Epithelioid (Spitz) Nevus

Barnhill RL. The spitzoid lesion: the importance of atypical variants and risk assessment. Am J Dermatopathol 2006; 28: 75–83.

Requena C, Requena L, Kutzner H, Sancez Yus E. Spitz nevus: a Clinicopathological study of 349 cases. Am J Dermatopathol 2009; 31: 107–116.

Wick MR, Patterson JW. Cutaneous melanocytic lesions: selected problem areas. Am J Clin Pathol 2005; 124 suppl: S52–S83.

Pigmented Spindle Cell Nevus

Barnhill RL. Malignant melanoma, dysplastic melanocytic nevi, and Spitz tumors. Histologic classification and characteristics. Clin Plast Surg 2000; 27: 331–360.

Barnhill RL, Barnhill MA, Berwick M, Michm MC Jr. The histologic spectrum of pigmented spindle cell nevus: a review of 120 cases with emphasis on atypical variants. Hum Pathol 1991; 22: 52–58.

Dal Pozzo V, Benelli C, Restano L, Gianotti R, Cesana BM. Clinical review of 247 case records of Spitz nevus (epithelioid cell and/or spindle cell nevus). Dermatology 1997; 194: 20–25.

Cellular Blue Nevus

Barnhill RL, Argenyi Z, Berwick M, Duray PH, Erickson L, Guitart J, Horenstein MG, Lowe L, Messina J, Paine S, Piepkorn MW, Prieto V, Rabkin M, Schmidt P, Selim A, Shea CR, Trotter MJ. Atypical cellular blue nevi (cellular blue nevi with atypical features): lack of consensus for diagnosis and distinction from cellular blue nevi and malignant melanoma ("malignant blue nevus"). Am J Surg Pathol 2008; 32: 36–44.

Mishima Y. Cellular blue nevus. Melanogenic activity and malignant transformation. Arch Dermatol 1970; 101: 104–110.

Temple-Camp CRE, Saxe N, King H. Benign and malignant cellular blue nevus. A clinicopathological study of 30 cases. Am J Dermatopathol 1988; 10: 289–296.

Deep Penetrating Nevus

Murali R, McCarthy SW, Scolyer RA. Blue nevi and related lesions: a review highlighting atypical and newly described variants, distinguishing features and diagnostic pitfalls. Adv Anat Pathol 2009; 16: 365–382.

Perez OG, Villoldo MS, Schroh R, Woscoff A. Deep penetrating nevus. J Eur Acad Dermatol Venereol 2009; 23: 703–704.

Robson A, Morley-Quante M, Hempel H, McKee PH, Calonje E. Deep penetrating naevus: clinicopathological study of 31 cases with further delineation of histologic features allowing distinction from other pigmented benign melanocytic lesions and melanoma. Histopathology 2003; 43: 529–537.

Balloon Cell Nevus

Goette DK, Doty, RD. Balloon cell nevus. Summary of the clinical and histologic characteristics. Arch Dermatol 1978; 114: 109–111.

Hashimoto K, Bale GF. An electron microscopic study of balloon cell nevus. Cancer 1972; 30: 530–540.

Martinez-Casimiro L, Sanchez-Carazo JL, Alegre V. Balloon cell naevus. J Eur Acad Dermatol Venereol 2009; 23: 236–237.

Smoller BR, Kindel S, McNutt NS, Gray MH, Hsu A. Balloon cell transformation in multiple dysplastic nevi. J Am Acad Dermatol 1991; 24: 290–292.

Recurrent Nevus

King R, Hayzen BA, Page RN, Googe PB, Zeagler D, Mihm MC Jr. Recurrent nevus phenomenon: a clinicopathologic study of 357 cases and histologic comparison with melanoma with regression. Mod Pathol 2009; 22: 611–617.

Park HK, Leonard DD, Arrington JH 3rd, Lund HZ. Recurrent melanocytic nevi: clinical and histologic review of 175 cases. J Am Acad Dermatol 1987; 17: 285–292.

Chapter 4

Seborrheic Keratoses

Izikson L, Sober AJ, Mihm MC Jr, Zembowicz A. Prevalence of melanoma clinically resembling seborrheic keratoses:

analysis of 9204 cases. Arch Dermatol 2002; 138: 1562–1566.

Noiles K, Vender R. Are all seborrheic keratoses benign? Review of the typical lesion and its variants. J Cutan Med Surg 2008; 12: 203–210.

Schwartz RA. Sign of Leser-Trelat. J Am Acad Dermatol 1996; 35: 88–95.

Inverted Follicular Keratoses

Ko CJ, Kim J, Phan J, Binder SW. Bcl-2 positive epidermal dendritic cells in inverted follicular keratoses but not squamous cell carcinomas or seborrheic keratoses. J Cutan Pathol 2006; 33: 498–501.

Mehregan AH. Inverted follicular keratoses is a distinct follicular tumor. Am J Dermatopathol 1983; 5: 467–470.

Reed RJ, Pulitzer DR. Inverted follicular keratoses and human papillomavirus. Am J Dermatopathol 1983; 5: 453–465.

Lichenoid Keratoses

Al-Hoqail IA, Crawford RI. Benign lichenoid keratoses with histologic features of mycosis fungoides: clinicopathologic description of a clinically significant histologic pattern. J Cutan Pathol 2002; 29: 291–294.

Morgan MB, Stevens GL, Switlyk S. Benign lichenoid keratoses: a clinical and pathologic reappraisal of 1040 cases. Am J Dermatopathol 2005; 27: 387–392.

Prieto VG, Casal M, McNutt NS. Lichen planus-like keratoses. A clinical and histological reexamination. Am J Surg Pathol 1993; 17: 259–263.

Actinic Keratoses

Davis DA, Donahue JP, Bost JE, Horn TD. The diagnostic concordance of actinic keratoses and squamous cell carcinoma. J Cutan Pathol 2005; 32: 546–551.

Roewert-Huber J, Stockfieth E, Kerl H. Pathology and pathobi-
ology of actinic (solar) keratoses – an update. Br J Dermatol
2007; 157 suppl 2: 18–20.

Rossi R, Mori M, Lotti T. Actinic keratoses. Int J Dermatol 2007;
46: 895–904.

Squamous Cell Carcinoma

Cassarino DS, Derienzo DP, Barr RJ. Cutaneous squamous cell
carcinoma: a comprehensive clinicopathologic classification.
Part one. J Cutan Pathol 2006; 33: 191–206.

Cassarino DS, Derienzo DP, Barr RJ. Cutaneous squamous cell
carcinoma: a comprehensive clinicopathologic classification.
Part two. J Cutan Pathol 2006; 33: 261–279.

Smoller BR. Squamous cell carcinoma: from precursor lesions to
high-risk variants. Mod Pathol 2006; 19 suppl 2: S88–S92.

Keratoacanthoma

Beham A, Regauer S, Soyer HP, Beham-Schmid C.
Keratoacanthoma: a clinically distinct variant of well differentiated squamous cell carcinoma. Adv Anat Pathol 1998;
5: 269–280.

Kane CL, Keehn CA, Smithberger E, Glass LF. Histopathology
of cutaneous squamous cell carcinoma and its variants. Semin
Cutan Med Surg 2004; 23: 54–61.

LeBoit PE. Can we understand keratoacanthoma? Am J
Dermatopathol 2002; 24: 166–168.

Basal Cell Carcinoma

Boulinguez S, Grison-Tabone C, Lamant L, Valmary S, Viraben R,
Bonnetblanc JM, Bedane C. Histologic evolution of recurrent
basal cell carcinoma and therapeutic implications for incom-
pletely excised lesions. Br J Dermatol 2004; 151: 623–626.

Miller SJ. Biology of basal cell carcinoma (Part 1). J Am Acad
Dermatol 1991; 24: 1–13.

Miller SJ. Biology of basal cell carcinoma (Part 2). J Am Acad
Dermatol 1991; 24: 161–175.

Saidanha G, Fletcher A, Slater DN. Basal cell carcinoma: a
dermatopathological and molecular biological update. Br J
Dermatol 2003; 148: 195–202.

Strutton GM. Pathological variants of basal cell carcinoma.
Australas J Dermatol 1997; 38 suppl 1: S31–35.

Extramammary Paget's Disease

Kanitakis J. Mammary and extramammary Paget's disease. J Eur
Acad Dermatol Venereol 2007; 21: 581–590.

Kohler S, Rouse RV, Smoller BR. The differential diagnosis of
Pagetoid cells in the epidermis. Mod Pathol 1998; 11: 79–92.

Chapter 5

Trichofolliculoma

Misago N, Kimura T, Toda S, Mori T, Narisawa Y. A
reevaluation of trichofolliculoma: the histopathological and
immunohistochemical features. Am J Dermatopathol 2010; 32:
154–161.

Plewig G. Sebaceous trichofolliculoma. J Cutan Pathol 1980; 7:
394–403.

Trichoepithelioma, Trichoadenoma, Trichoblastoma

Brooke JD, Fitzpatrick JE, Golitz LE. Papillary mesenchymal
bodies: a histologic finding useful in differentiating trichoepitheliomas from basal cell carcinomas. J Am Acad Dermatol
1989; 21: 523–528.

LeBoit PE. Trichoblastoma, basal cell carcinoma, and follicular differentiation: what should we trust? Am J Dermatopathol 2003; 25: 260–263.

Rahbari H, Mehregan A, Pinkus H. Trichoadenoma of Nikolowski. J Cutan Pathol 1977; 4: 90–98.

Pilomatricoma

Hardisson D, Linares MD, Cuevas-Santos J, Contreras F. Pilomatrix carcinoma: a clinicopathologic study of six cases and review of the literature. Am J Dermatopathol 2001; 23: 394–401.

Julian CG, Bowers PW. A clinical review of 209 pilomatricomas. J Am Acad Dermatol 1998; 39: 191–195.

Lan MY, Lan MC, Ho CY, Li WY, Lin CZ. Pilomatricoma of the head and neck: a retrospective review of 179 cases. Arch Otolaryngol Head Neck Surg 2003; 129: 1327–1330.

Trichilemmoma

Brownstein MH. Trichilemmoma. Benign follicular tumor or viral wart? Am J Dermatopathol 1980; 2: 229–231.

Hidayat AA, Font RL. Trichilemmoma of eyelid and eyebrow. A clinicopathologic study of 31 cases. Arch Ophthalmol 1980; 98: 844–847.

Rohwedder A, Keminer O, Hendricks C, Schaller J. Detection of HPV DNA in trichilemmomas by polymerase chain reaction. J Med Virol 1997; 51: 119–125.

Tellechea O, Reis JP, Baptista AP. Desmoplastic trichilemmoma. Am J Dermatopathol 1992; 14: 107–114.

Proliferating Trichilemmal Tumor

Folpe AL, Reisenauer AK, Mentzel T, Rutten A, Solomon AR. Proliferating trichilemmal tumors: clinicopathologic evaluation is a guide to biologic behavior. J Cutan Pathol 2003; 30: 492–498.

Satyaprakash AK, Sheehan DJ, Sangueza OP. Proliferating trichilemmal tumors: a review of the literature. Dermatol Surg 2007; 33: 1102–1108.

Fibrofolliculoma

Starink TM, Brownstein MH. Fibrofolliculoma: solitary and multiple types. J Am Acad Dermatol 1987; 17: 493–496.
Welsch MJ, Krunic A, Medenica MM. Birt-Hogg-Dube syndrome. Int J Dermatol 2005; 44: 668–673.

Trichodiscoma

Vincent A, Farley M, Chan E, James WD. Birt-Hogg-Dube syndrome: a review of the literature and the differential diagnosis of firm facial papules. J Am Acad Dermatol 2003; 49: 698–705.
Welsch MJ, Krunic A, Medenica MM. Birt-Hogg-Dube syndrome. Int J Dermatol 2005; 44: 668–673.

Tumor of the Follicular Infundibulum

Abbas O, Mahalingam M. Tumor of the follicular infundibulum: an epidermal reaction pattern? Am J Dermatopathol 2009; 31: 626–633.
Cribier B, Grosshans E. Tumor of the follicular infundibulum: a clinicopathologic study. J Am Acad Dermatol 1995; 33: 979–984.
Weyers W, Horster S, Diaz-Cascajo C. Tumor of follicular infundibulum is basal cell carcinoma. Am J Dermatopathol 2009; 31: 634–641.

Nevus Sebaceus of Jadassohn

Cribier B, Scivener Y, Grosshans E. Tumors arising in nevus sebaceus: a study of 596 cases. J Am Acad Dermatol 2000; 42: 263–268.

Eisen DB, Michael DJ. Sebaceous lesions and their associated syndromes. Part 1. J Am Acad Dermatol 2009; 61: 549–560.
Prioleau PG, Santa Cruz DJ. Sebaceous gland neoplasia. J Cutan Pathol 1984; 11: 396–414.

Sebaceous Hyperplasia

Eisen DB, Michael DJ. Sebaceous lesions and their associated syndromes. Part 1. J Am Acad Dermatol 2009; 61: 549–560.

Sebaceous Adenoma

Abbas O, Mahalingam M. Cutaneous sebaceous neoplasms as markers of Muir-Torre syndrome: a diagnostic algorithm. J Cutan Pathol 2009; 36: 613–619.
Abbott JJ, Hernandez-Rios P, Amirkhan RH, Hoang MP. Cystic sebaceous neoplasms in Muir-Torre syndrome. Arch Pathol Lab Mcd 2003; 127: 614–617.
Eisen DB, Michael DJ. Sebaceous lesions and their associated syndromes. Part 1. J Am Acad Dermatol 2009; 61: 549–560.

Sebaceoma (Sebaceous Epithelioma)

Eisen DB, Michael DJ. Sebaceous lesions and their associated syndromes. Part 1. J Am Acad Dermatol 2009; 61: 549–560.
Misago N, Mihara I, Ansai S, Narisawa Y. Sebaceoma and related neoplasms with sebaceous differentiation: a clinicopathologic study of 30 cases. Am J Dermatopathol 2002; 24: 294–304.
Troy JL, Ackerman AB. Sebaceoma. A distinctive benign neoplasm of adnexal epithelium differentiating toward sebaceous cells. Am J Dermatopathol 1984; 6: 7–13.

Sebaceous Carcinoma

Pereira PR, Odashiro AN, Rodrigues-Reyes AA, Correa ZM, de Souza Filho JP, Burnier MN Jr. Histopathological review of sebaceous carcinoma of the eyelid. J Cutan Pathol 2005; 32: 496–501.

Prioleau PG, Santa Cruz DJ. Sebaceous gland neoplasia. J Cutan Pathol 1984; 11: 396–414.

Muir–Torre Syndrome

Abbott JJ, Hernandez-Rios P, Amirkhan RH, Hoang MP. Cystic sebaceous neoplasms in Muir-Torre syndrome. Arch Pathol Lab Med 2003; 127: 614–617.

Ponti G, Ponz de Leon M. Muir-Torre syndrome. Lancet Oncol 2005; 6: 980–987.

Schwartz RA, Torre DP. The Muir-Torre syndrome: a 25 year retrospective. J Am Acad Dermatol 1995; 33: 90–104.

Chapter 6

Eccrine Poroma/Porocarcinoma

Brown CW Jr, Dy LC. Eccrine porocarcinoma. Dermatol Ther 2008; 21: 433–438.

Pylyser K, De Wolf-Peeteres C, Marien K. The histology of eccrine poromas: a study of 14 cases. Dermatologica 1983; 167: 243–249.

Robson A, Greene J, Ansari N, Kim B, Seed PT, McKee PH, Calonje E. Eccrine porocarcinoma (malignant eccrine poroma): a clinicopathologic study of 69 cases. Am J Surg Pathol 2001; 25: 710–720.

Hidradenoma/Hidradenocarcinoma

Crowson AN, Magro CM, Mihm MC. Malignant eccrine neoplasms. Mod Pathol 2006; 19 suppl 2: S93–S126.

Hernandez-Perez E, Cestoni-Parducci R. Nodular hidradenoma and hidradenocarcinoma. A 10 year review. J Am Acad Dermatol 1985; 12: 15–20.

Souvatzidis P, Sbano P, Mandato F, Fimiani M, Castelli
A. Malignant nodular hidradenoma of the skin: report of
seven cases. J Eur Acad Dermatol Venerol 2008; 22:
549–554.

Dermal Duct Tumor

Faure M, Colomb D. Dermal duct tumor. J Cutan Pathol 1979; 6:
317–322.
Hanau D, Grosshans E, Laplanche G. A complex poroma-like
adnexal adenoma. Am J Dermatopathol 1984; 6: 567–572.
Winkelmann RK, McLeod WA. The dermal duct tumor. Arch
Dermatol 1966; 94: 50–55.

Spiradenoma/Spiradenocarcinoma

Argenyi ZB, Nguyen AV, Balogh K, Sears JK, Whitaker DC.
Malignant eccrine spiradenoma. A clinicopathologic study. Am
J Dermatopathol 1992; 14: 381–390.
Baes H. Eccrine spiradenoma. Acta Derm Venereol 1967; 47:
447–450.
Cooper PH, Frierson HF Jr, Morrison AG. Malignant transfor-
mation of eccrine spiradenoma. Arch Dermatol 1985; 121:
1445–1448.
Mambo NC. Eccrine spiradenoma: clinical and pathologic study
of 49 tumors. J Cutan Pathol 1983; 10: 312–320.

Cylindroma

Gerretsen SL, van der Putte SC, Deenstra W, van Vloten WA.
Cutaneous cylindroma with malignant transformation. Cancer
1993; 72: 1618–1623.
Lian F, Cockerell CJ. Cutaneous appendage tumors: familial cylin-
dromatosis and associated tumors update. Adv Dermatol 2005;
21: 217–234.

Syringoma

Patrizi A, Neri I, Marzaduri S, Varotti E, Passarini B. Syringoma: a review of twenty-nine cases. Acta Derm Venereol 1998; 78: 460–462.

Pruzan DL, Esterly NB, Prose NS. Eruptive syringoma. Arch Dermatol 1989; 125: 1119–1120.

Saitoh A, Ohtake N, Fukuda S, Tamaki K. Clear cells of eccrine glands in a patient with clear cell syringoma associated with diabetes mellitus. Am J Dermatopathol 1993; 15: 166–168.

Chondroid Syringoma

Mentzel T, Requena L, Kaddu S, Soares de Aleida LM, Sangueza OP, Kutzner H. Cutaneous myoepithelial neoplasms: clinicopathologic and immunohistochemical study of 20 cases suggesting a continuous spectrum ranging from benign mixed tumor of the skin to cutaneous myoepithelioma and myoepithelial carcinoma. J Cutan Pathol 2003; 30: 294–302.

Microcystic Adnexal Carcinoma

Friedman PM, Friedman RH, Jiang SB, Nouri K, Amonette R, Robins P. Microcystic adnexal carcinoma: collaborative series review and update. J Am Acad Dermatol 1999; 41: 225–231.

Ohtsuka H, Nagamatsu S. Microcystic adnexal carcinoma: review of 51 Japanese patients. Dermatology 2002; 204: 190–193.

Wetter R, Goldstein GD. Microcystic adnexal carcinoma: a diagnostic and therapeutic challenge. Dermatol Ther 2008; 21: 452–458.

Eccrine Nevus

Requena L, Sangueza OP. Cutaneous vascular anomalies. Part 1. Hamartomas, malformations and dilation of preexisting vessels. J Am Acad Dermatol 1997; 37: 523–549.

Sulica RL, Kao GF, Sulica VI, Penneys NS. Eccrine angiomatous hamartoma (nevus): immunohistochemical findings and review of the literature. J Cutan Pathol 1994; 21: 71–75.

Syringofibroadenoma

Alli N, Polat M, Cinar SL, Kulacoglu S. Eccrine syringofibroadenoma. Eur J Dermatol 2008; 18: 478–479.

Takeda H, Mitsuhashi Y, Hayashi M, Kondo S. Eccrine syringofibroadenoma: case report and review of the literature. J Eur Acad Dermatol Venereol 2001; 15: 147–149.

Mucinous Syringometaplasia

Kappel TJ, Abenoza P. Mucinous syringometaplasia. A case report with review of the literature. Am J Dermatopathol 1993; 15: 562–567.

Trotter MJ, Stevens PJ, Smith NP. Mucinous syringometaplasia-a case report and review of the literature. Clin Exp Dermatol 1995; 20: 42–45.

Papillary Eccrine Adenoma

Mizuoka H, Senzaki H, Shikata N, Uemura Y, Tsubura A. Papillary eccrine adenoma: immunohistochemical study and literature review. J Cutan Pathol 1998; 25: 59–64.

Smith KJ, Skelton HG, Holland TT. Recent advances and controversies concerning adnexal neoplasms. Dermatol Clin 1992; 10: 117–160.

Hidradenoma Papilliferum

Fernancez-Acenero MJ, Sanchez TA, Sanchez MC, Requena L. Ectopic hidradenoma papilliferum: a case report and literature review. Am J Dermatopathol 2003; 25: 176–178.

Goette DK. Hidradenoma papilliferum. J Am Acad Dermatol 1988; 19: 133–135.

Virgili A, Marzola A, Corazza M. Vulvar hidradenoma papilliferum. A review of 10.5 years experience. J Reprod Med 2000; 45: 616–618.

Syringocystadenoma Papilliferum

Cribier B, Scrivener Y, Grosshans E. Tumors arising in nevus sebaceus: a study of 56 cases. J Am Acad Dermatol 2000; 42: 263–268.

Rammen-Rommani S, Fezaa B, Chelbi E, Sammoun MR, Ben Jilani SB, Zermani R. Syringocystadenoma papilliferum: report of 8 cases. Pathologica 2006; 98: 178–180.

Aggressive Digital Papillary Adenocarcinoma

Duke WH, Sherrod TT, Lupton GP. Aggressive digital papillary adenocarcinoma (aggressive digital papillary adenoma and adenocarcinoma revisited). Am J Surg Pathol 2000; 24: 775–784.

Kao GF, Helwig EB, Graham JH. Aggressive digital papillary adenoma and adenocarcinoma. A clinicopathologic study of 57 patients, with histochemical, immunopathological, and ultrastructural observations. J Cutan Pathol 1987; 14: 129–146.

Chapter 7

Merkel Cell Carcinoma

Andea AA, Coit DG, Amin B, Busam KJ. Merkel cell carcinoma: histologic features and prognosis. Cancer 2008; 113: 2549–2558.

Busam KJ, Jungbluth AA, Rekthman N, Coit D, Pulitzer M, Bini J, Arora R, Hanson NC, Tassello JA, Frosina D, Moore P,

Chang Y. Merkel cell polyomavirus expression in Merkel cell carcinomas and its absence in combined tumors and pulmonary neuroendocrine carcinomas. Am J Surg Pathol 2009; 33: 1378–1385.

Duncavage EJ, Le BM, Wang D, Pfeifer JD. Merkel cell polyomavirus: a specific marker for Merkel cell carcinoma in histologically similar tumors. Am J Surg Pathol 2009; 33: 1771–1777.

Pulitzer MP, Amin BD, Busam KJ. Merkel cell carcinoma: review. Adv Anat Pathol 2009; 16: 135–144.

Index

Printed in the United States of America